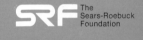

YOUR MONEY OR YOUR LIFE

Rx for the Medical Market Place

YOUR MONEY
OR YOUR LIFE

Rx for the Medical Market Place

By RICHARD KUNNES, M.D.

DODD, MEAD & COMPANY

NEW YORK

ISBN: 0-396-06422-1
Library of Congress Catalog Card Number: 72-169733

Printed in the United States of America
by The Cornwall Press, Inc., Cornwall, N.Y.

Prologue

What makes someone want to be a physician? For myself, I always wanted the money and the prestige. In addition, however, and even more importantly, I wanted to be of use to others. Medicine seemed to meet these three criteria of money, prestige, and service. In substance, however, it met only the first two. How could I be comfortable with the privilege and power that comes from being a physician, without the rationalization that I was serving people?

At least in the beginning, the fact that medicine wasn't all it was alleged to be, that the myth of medicine was nothing like the reality of the madness of medicine wasn't all that significant to me. I knew there were problems in the medical system just as there were problems in the educational and the economic systems. The problems were seen as mild, and even sometimes major, aberrations in an otherwise worthwhile, democratic society. I don't mean to give the impression that I started my medical training and career in a state of total naïveté. By the first year of college, while still in my teens, I was in political demonstrations and was occasionally arrested. I had some sense that America had another side, but not enough to realize that one couldn't practice medicine here without being an oppressor.

How did I finally come to such a realization? While I can't reconstruct all the reasons which lead me to this position, I can mention a few:

The expanding war in Viet Nam contributed to my new awareness. In large part it was the daily, unending, and unnecessary civilian and military casualties that moved me. Military might was being converted into a massive medical problem, and the war was not going to be ended or the dying stopped by practicing medicine—of any kind.

My medical training at a number of the most prestigious university medical centers, while supposedly the best available, was mindless and alienating. There was little that had any connection with the medical necessities of our time. Heads were separate from bodies and both were separate from people. That is, we learned about organs and not people, about disease and not health. Medical care had more to do with professional concepts than with human concern. The theory didn't fit the practice, and the practice which was worth anything to medical students was usually of little value to patients.

Introduction

The American health-care system functions within, and is a part and product of, the American economic system. The problems, faults, and contradictions of the economic system are inherent in the health-care system but much more serious in this context. It will be the purpose of this book to highlight, analyze, and evaluate these problems, faults, and contradictions.

The American health-care system has been dominated by the American Medical Association. The AMA has said time after time that Americans receive the best medical care in the world. The truth is that only relatively well-off Americans receive the best health care in the world. The rest of us have to live with the following facts:

1. The United States is ranked 22nd in life expectancy.
2. The United States is ranked 18th in infant mortality.
3. The United States is ranked 15th in the ratio of hospital beds to population.
4. 20 per cent of all military draftees are rejected for medical reasons.

5. Only 60 per cent of United States hospitals are accredited, and almost 3 million patients a year are treated in unaccredited hospitals.
6. In New York City alone, 71 per cent of all nursing positions are vacant.
7. There are fewer doctors on a per capita basis today than at the turn of the century.

In spite of the scandalous figures listed above, the American health-care system is the most expensive in the world, and yet delivers shockingly few services. In the fiscal year 1969, the United States spent an estimated $60 billion for health purposes. One would think that this huge sum (more expenditures per capita than for any country in the world), guaranteed a decent system. However, were it not for the importation of often poorly trained foreign medical manpower, our fragile health system would certainly collapse. And yet despite the fact that we are woefully short of physicians and medical schools, at least a score of the ninety-eight United States medical schools are near closing for lack of funds, and thousands of academically qualified students can't get funds to attend medical school.

This situation has angered both patients and some professionals. As a physician practicing within the American medical system, I have been increasingly appalled as more and more deficiencies come to light. In July of 1969, in an effort to dramatize the inadequacies of the health system, I went before the AMA convention, publicly burned my AMA membership card, and presented a statement to the AMA House of Delegates, the ruling body of American medicine.

The assembled doctors were more than a little angry at the statement. Some threw heavy glass ashtrays at me—all in the name of preserving our American health system with all its faults intact.

In response to the ashtray throwing, an articulate health consumer, said:

"Medical care in this country is like a pay toilet. You take a biological necessity and then charge to have it satisfied. Well, let me tell you, there's a lot of people who can't afford the price of admission anymore. And these people are getting madder'n hell at having to crawl under the john door, just to meet their needs. They're tired of wallowing in all that crap. And soon they're going to rip that door off its hinges."

Well, what are some of the reasons for this outpouring of venom directed toward doctors, even by other doctors? One of the reasons is their arrogance and professionalism—what some have called "white-coat privileges." Let me give you an example of professional arrogance and white-coat privilege:

An auto-accident victim, suffering from a chest injury, was brought into a hospital's emergency room in Philadelphia. An intern examined the patient, sent him to X-ray, and called the chest-surgery resident on call. In the X-ray room, the patient became increasingly frightened about his condition. The chief of the chest-surgery service, who happened to be nearby, interjected himself and told the patient to "shut up and show the proper respect." This of course only frightened the patient more. The chief of the chest-surgery service, without examining the patient, *ordered him out of the hospital.* The intern and X-ray technician managed to calm down the patient to the point where the chief of the service agreed to allow him to stay in the hospital to complete his X-ray. The X-ray did indeed reveal a serious injury. The chest-surgery resident, however, by this time feeling as insulted and as put upon as did the chief of the service, refused to see the patient. Another chest-surgery resident had to be called from home to treat the patient.

Unfortunately the current anger directed at doctors isn't caused just by their professional arrogance. The causes are deeper and the responsibilities for the glaring deficiencies in health care go much further than individual doctors or even the AMA.

For example, New York City, because of its large, diverse, sophisticated population and problems, often has to confront issues before they become issues in other areas of the country. Health care in New York City is no exception: what problems exist in medical care throughout the country are then multiplied. The Blue Cross-Blue Shield system in New York City recently asked for an 83 per cent rate increase. Patients, and even some physicians, were outraged by this rate hike. The State Insurance Department of New York held hearings on the insurance premium increase. In an attempt to alert people to the devastating effect of rising health-care costs, a group of us illegally took control of the hearings and were arrested. Fortunately, the Mayor was sufficiently aroused to file suit against Blue Cross. While we were promptly released, Blue Cross was granted its requested fee increase.

Needless to say, the health system and its supporters are a little up tight about any serious criticism. But my differences with the AMA and its corporate and professional associates are not simply isolated ideological or theoretical differences, but life and death differences. Whoever controls health care in this country literally has the power to determine life and death for millions of people. Should this power rest in the hands of selfish corporate and professional interests?

These interests have developed a technically advanced country that can land a man on the moon and explode hydrogen bombs, but can't provide efficient ambulance service to take someone to the hospital.

What has created this sorry state of affairs? Who is to blame? And what can be done about it?

Contents

PART ONE

THE MEDICAL MARKET PLACE

I

Medical Imperialism: The Medical Profession

BACKGROUND

Men who prescribe medicine of which they know little, to cure diseases of which they know less, in human beings of whom they know nothing.

—Voltaire

In medicine, the doctors control knowledge. They also control who is admitted to the profession. The work situation for other health workers is determined by doctors and the procedures doctors want carried out, rather than by consumers or communities. Dr. Victor Fuchs, health policy researcher, said in *Medical Economics that* "though the physician may get less than 15% of the health care dollar (net income) his authority over hospitalization and drugs makes him the controlling influence with respect to 90% of it!"

The purpose of this book is not to condemn individual doctors, but rather to focus blame on the system that encourages them to act the way they do. In a profiteering private practice the MD is the focus and immediate source of serious conflicts of interest. He is either forced by the limitations of the patient's pocketbook to compromise and to settle for paltry palliatives that fall far short of what is medically possible, or to charge all the patient will bear—or both.

The setting where doctors practice is the medical market place, the infrastructure of the health system. It tends to be both visible and public. This book will also deal with the medical-industrial complex (MIC), the suprastructure. The MIC is often invisible, private, and unaccountable. It manipulates behind the scenes the quality and quantity of health care delivered.

Why has the medical profession clung to "rugged individualism," cottage industries, and old-fashioned entrepreneurial practices, i.e., why have doctors lagged behind all other segments of the economy, failing to evolve to a more advanced form of capitalism? Studies have shown that only United States Supreme Court judges outrank physicians in general prestige and status. The profession's conservatism is enhanced by its being the most lucrative of all the professions. Professional conservatism encourages conformity, and vice versa, and thus selects against the "great unwashed"—the poor, the black, and the Puerto Rican.

Apparently MD's have a vested interest in an entrepreneurial system, under which they have total, unaccountable control of the medical market place. They are the arbiters of quality and ethics. These MD's are also derived from the most conservative elements of society. Indeed, most MD's today come from families of MD's. It is the most tradition-loaded of all the professions. For the last 100 years, MD's have gained the highest status, prestige, and compensation, and thus have the greatest stake in the existing system; they thus resist any change which might interfere with their status and power.

The evolution of the economy had its effect on medical care. It meant that the MD couldn't act much longer as an isolated entrepreneur, but rather needed nurses, aides, secretaries, technicians, hospitals, government agencies, and officials at all levels, as well as laboratories, equipment, and specialization. This meant that many MD's would have to assume an increasing role more akin to a bureaucratic executive, rather than an independent businessman. However, while the business world was liberalized into bureaucratic corporations, the MD resisted, fighting for his individualism —which meant fighting for his privileges, profits, and prerogatives.

The doctor in one sense did have the most to lose compared to all other business sectors and professions. Some claim that the medical profession is far more "concerned with resisting change than guiding." But guiding it or controlling it is only the liberal side of the capitalistic coin. Resisting change is conservative; guiding and controlling it is liberal—neither of which solves the conflict of service to humanity versus making a profit, on a fee-for-service basis. The doctors' need to get paid conflicts with the patient's need to get well. And whether one takes a conservative or liberal approach, the basic profit system, with its inherent conflicts with health services, will prevail. Increasing incomes have allowed MD's to reach new social status and strata. The stratification and status are used further by the MD to insure and promote his control over the patient-consumer population and the medical market place. Increasing incomes and use of them for political purposes have enhanced the position and strength of the medical profession further, particularly when in alliance with the medical-industrial complex.

No other profession is so literally vital as is medicine. The medical profession has intimidated the public to gain its status and prestige. The profession has bought political power with the highest lobbying fees in history. No other segment of, or profession in, society so completely guarantees its members so much wealth, status, and power. No other segment of society has been so successful from a self-interested point, politically, socially, and economically. The medical profession and now the medical-industrial complex have the greatest marketing gimmick of all time—life versus death and disease. Thus they, the profession and the MIC, are in a position to blackmail their way to a point powerful enough to shape the system to suit them profitably, even if it means the neglect of the health of millions of people.

Most medical students come from the upper middle classes and thus most strive to work in upper-middle-class neighborhoods, not only because it's more profitable and prestigious, but because the young doctors are more comfortable with the clientele from their own economic, social, and racial backgrounds. The racism instilled in these students from their white upper-middle-class upbringing makes it difficult for them to establish warm, supportive, mature relationships with people "below" them in class and race. (See Appendix A for an example of an attempt to challenge such familial and educational background.) Dr. Richard Weinerman of Yale University, School of Medicine, notes that the isolation of such upbringing produces considerable ignorance about the less fortunate and more oppressed segments of our population. He notes that even when the students see patients in their clinical work "they are seeing their patients in a frame far more flattering than normal. They have never seen or smelled bad housing. They know nothing of the reality of bad diets, of broken homes, of unemployment, of what it means when the breadwinner is sent to the hospital for a long stay, of the thousand and one things never seen at the hospital bedside or in the dispensary." And the other side of it is that such ignorance is encouraged and enhanced. Quality patient care does not mesh with the teaching institutions' priorities of research and treatment of relatively acute diseases—all within the confines and control of the hospital.

THE PHYSICIAN

The training of physicians is time consuming and tradition bound. Tradition is instilled into the medical student by fear: fear of failure to pass a course, to get a good recommendation for an internship, or to gain hospital staff privileges. Of course, tradition is also instilled by way of example. But regardless, if the medical student doesn't admire his preceptor, he at least fears him and one way or another will be forced to emulate him.

The length of time, strain, deprivation, and little or no money associated with medical training can only be dehumanizing, can only create an emotional and economic dependency on the rulers of the health system, and breed cynicism. Medical training used to be divided into preclinical and clinical years. It's now called the precynical and cynical years.

There are many factors that create this cynicism. Long years of emotional and economic deprivation make the new physician's appetite for money all the greater—by any means necessary. Part of the physician's concern about his income is to make up and pay back loans he incurred during his long years of training. During the time it takes to build up a practice he also must have funds to pay for financing expensive equipment, furniture, paying nurses, aides, secretaries, and accountants. At the time of the completion of my residency I was $15,000 in debt.

The young resident has noticed that patients die routinely because of doctor and nurse shortages. There is not enough manpower to observe the patient even when he is in the hospital. When patients are brought into the hospital half dead because of a delay in seeking treatment, or because of an inability to afford a physician's or clinic's fees, the young doctor begins to understand how irrelevant his medical education is under such circumstances. If patients, because of geographic, manpower, or financial inaccessibility of services seek treatment only when it's too late, it doesn't matter how skilled he is—it's too late and it becomes clear that it will take something more than a "revised curriculum in biochemistry" to deal with these issues. The fact that the only responses to such issues as mass patient neglect have been either curriculum reform or changes in insurance plans adds to one's cynicism.

Drug companies lavish expensive books, black medical bags, stethoscopes, and mountains of free drugs on medical students. While the medical student's ego might be expanded by the hundreds of dollars per year spent on him by slick drug companies, he is also aware that he cannot legally use the drugs. He increasingly realizes that because inflated drug prices also result from the drug companies' advertising campaigns that are directed at medical students, many patients cannot adhere to an expensive drug regiment.

Students also learn to accept orders unquestioningly. When

their superiors order unnecessary tests or are unnecessarily rough with the patient, students know better than to question. Aside from the cynicism is the conveyance of an image of the physician as authoritarian, masculine, and white. On the other hand, "patients are seen as weak-willed, self-centered and unreasonably demanding."

The cynicism, the need to adhere to authority, the contradiction between superficial humanitarian concern and substantive economic interests combine to produce a disproportionate number of emotionally disturbed MD's, in a profession that requires the greatest emotional stability. Studies show that MD's have the highest suicide rate.

The entire educational process, moreover, encourages a sense of personal inadequacy. During his internship, the young intern is often given undue responsibility, which he just isn't equipped to handle. This sense of inadequacy, as well as social, economic, and academic dependency, is encouraged, as it produces less chance of rebellion, facilitates a hierarchical structure, and eases the conflict between the superficial meaning of professional ethics and the substance of professional economics.

The castrating dominance and authority of medical institutions is further exacerbated by the medical student's increasing dependence on his wife's income from her working. He becomes accustomed to the idea that everything and everyone is sacrificed for his education, career, and profession. In an attempt to overcome his dependency and sense of castration, he is driven to gain an earlier and greater profit when he sets up his practice and is thus motivated to be as exploitative as possible—just as the institution where he worked exploited him as an intern and resident.

Dr. Alan Gregg, a renowned medical educator, said, ". . .

a physician is so surrounded by frightened patients, adoring families and obsequious nurses that he will not brook criticism by God or Man." This is the result of the professional control of the medical system. The AMA's own study of medical students found them to be of "above average IQ but intellectually lacking." That is, they weren't intellectually curious; they didn't question or probe or ask embarrassing and relevant questions. It is to the advantage of a medical school and of the AMA to deny admission to medical school the intellectually curious student. Future students almost naturally conform before even coming to medical school. The training of the physician is the mechanical training for a vocation and not the intellectual training of a humanitarian and skilled scientist. Training emphasizes technology and technique, all of which adds to the mystification and professionalization process and all of which discourages freedom of thought and action.

Medical education more often than not satiates the medical student's appetite for knowledge, as well as his curiosity and imagination, rather than stimulates it. Again this has an economic role in that it fosters dependency and creates a greater sense of ignorance in the medical student and an often unearned awe for his teachers, all of which greases an authoritarian system. If it does this to the student you can imagine what it does to the patient. The emphasis on memorization of irrelevant facts and minutiae has been castigated by one physician who said, ". . . facts are soon forgotten and in any case, the so-called facts of today often are the discarded myths of tomorrow." But the incredible burden of memorization is another method of eliminating competition, enhancing mystification, and thus controlling the medical market.

The drop in the quality of medical students in recent years

(as shown in a 1968 study by the American Association of Medical Colleges) is in part related to the emphasis by the profession on technology and limitations on intellectual freedom, especially when compared with other professions. The drop in quality and the continuation of intellectual narrowness are particularly ominous, in view of the fact that quality medical care is increasingly determined by a vast range of intellectually relevant political, economic, social, and emotional issues. Training for medicine is so strenuous that it allows the student, interne, or resident little time for any outside interests. Thus it is easier to control and inculcate him, as though he were in a monastery, accountable for his every word, thought, and deed. The parallels to religious training are not coincidental (cf. "laity" used in both religion and medicine, as is "mysticism").

During the Depression even physicians experienced a drop in income. The profession felt that it could preserve its financial status by the elimination of potential competition, by limiting the supply of physicians, or in the words of a medical researcher, ". . . commit professional birth control." In their efforts at professional birth control the profession has been highly successful. Fifty to sixty years ago there was one medical school graduate for every twenty thousand persons. Today that ratio is closer to one for every thirty thousand persons. Today seven countries, including the Soviet Union, have a higher proportion of doctors to population than does the United States. Thanks to this "birth control," there are now shortages in every part of the country and in every specialty. Rural areas have only one-third the practitioners of urban areas on a per capita basis and even the urban areas themselves are grossly understaffed. Just to bring all parts of the country up to the levels of the vastly understaffed urban areas would require an additional 100,000 MD's—now. And that says nothing of the number needed for optimal levels of health. Such shortages are equally as acute —and fatal—in all areas of health—for dentists, nurses, psychologists, social workers, technicians, aides, researchers, and so forth. There is, for example, a fantastic shortage of dentists, with quality of care and quantity of need directly proportionate to the ability to pay. In other words, the poorer you are, the lower the quality and the higher the need. Today, one in six Americans have never gone to a dentist.

Aside from shortages of health personnel, what little man and woman power exist is grossly maldistributed. Health reporter Selig Greenberg notes that "In Massachusetts there is one MD for every 550 persons; in Mississippi the average is one for every 1300. In Connecticut there is one graduate nurse for every 270 persons; in Kentucky the figure is one for every 860." Again, let us not forget that in spite of the better figures in Connecticut and Massachusetts, both states are desperately in need of more MD's, more nurses, more health professionals. There are openings literally for every category of health worker at every hospital in the country. The shortage is especially acute among psychiatrists. In New York City there is one psychiatrist for every 6500 persons; in Alabama there is one for every 65,000 persons, and yet NYC is desperately short of psychiatrists.

Even the recent increase in medical schools by no means represents a net gain. About four thousand physicians die every year and a number of others retire from practice or go into research or industry. Even if there were no changes in population in the last fifty years, manpower problems would still be exacerbated by the economic impetus to specialization and the attendant multiple referrals. The patient who saw one MD for his chest pain thirty years ago, now sees two or three, all of whom have more equipment, requiring manpower to develop and run—and all this, naturally, inflates costs. Increasingly sophisticated patients in an age of alienation, anxiety, and exploitation expect and need more time from the physician, not less. This places the patient in direct conflict with the MD's economic need to see patients quickly and is one reason for the great rise in malpractice suits.

For an example of the crisis in the manpower situation, a family needs not just a single personal family physician but rather, as a result of specialization, requires an entire personal health cadre—composed of internists, pediatricians, obstetricians, psychiatrists, and so on. What one MD used to do is now done by four or five, not to mention all the ancillary professionals needed. It's on a basis of health cadre, rather than on a single MD, to patient ratio that we must determine manpower needs.

The doctor shortage has meant decreased accessibility of physicians and an increase in crisis care, because of delays in seeking treatment. This produces an overflow in emergency rooms and consequently an increase in mortality and morbidity. As an indication of our shortage of physicians and health personnel, the District of Columbia in 1964 had the highest ratio in the United States of MD's to patients (excluding federally employed MD's) and yet had the highest neonatal mortality rate and second highest infant mortality in the country—only Mississippi was worse in this rate.

It is clear that medical schools no longer attract the cream of the crop. In the 20's and 30's one had to have nearly straight "A's" to gain medical school admission. Medical schools now accept a large proportion of "B" and "C" students. While there is no indication that new physicians are any less competent than their predecessors, the standards of medical schools have declined.

Shortages of MD's and inaccessibility of services result in delays in seeking and receiving quality service. It is hardly surprising therefore that people will go to their local pharmacist for advice and wind up taking Tums for their heart attacks.

More and more MD's occupy their time on boards of directors of industrial, nonhealth related concerns. Thus the number of licensed MD's is really no indication of the number of available, practicing MD's, and those who are practicing aren't necessarily practicing in the geographic or specialty area of greatest need.

The AMA is a monopoly and an elite group and functions as such. The economics of monopoly control and its consequent behavior of exploitation apply to the AMA. Thus as a monopoly class, the AMA has worked hard to ensure manpower shortages. Some of the following mechanisms are applicable.

No other profession dominates its professional education and presumes to set limits to the number of recruits to its calling to the degree that the medical profession does. To control educational standards, to limit class size and school construction, as well as tuition aid, the number of practicing physicians has purposefully been kept small. The smaller the supply, the greater the demand and the more the physician can charge. The higher the doctor's fee, the more money available to maintain the highest paid and largest lobby both in the national as well as state capitals throughout the country. The profession has attempted to consolidate its control at every opportunity; in the educational arena in medical schools, in hospital and training programs, licensing and accreditation, hospital admitting privileges, medical society membership, editorial control of professional health journals, political liaisons with tobacco, drug, insurance, hospital suppliers and contractors and governmental agencies—funding and regulatory. And all this activity takes place on the state and national levels.

Certain mechanisms have been devised to create manpower shortage. These are:

1. *The need for physical, financial, emotional, and intellectual stamina.* This is an artificial criteria by which to select future physicians. Medical education need not to be strenuous, physically, emotionally, financially, or intellectually. It certainly need not be so time consuming (i.e., twelve years). The twelve years of training alone make for an artificial selection criteria. Such criteria create artificial shortages of physicians, which is one reason why the shortages exist. Many doctors feel that the amount of medical material taught only adds to the mystique and professionalism of the physician, but not to his quality.

Unending periods of study mean the student must forego much needed humanizing personal and familial relationships. This lack not only tends to make the training more dehumanizing but leaves the student with only one significant relationship—between himself and the profession, its needs and demands. Even dehumanization serves an economic role. After all, there is no objective reason or financial motive for the physician to be interested in people—just the opposite. The less interested the physician is, the quicker his examinations and visits; the more patients he sees, the more money he can make.

The formidable and rigorous training process is itself a prolonged screening period wherein the student or young intern is carefully observed, not so much to insure that he dispenses quality care, but that he adheres to the rules and regulations of his profession. Only the most conforming and abiding survive this screening process. Rigorous training and screening not only enforce conformity, but frighten away a good deal of competition. The degree of conformity required is quite pervasive. It begins at the time a person first thinks of becoming a physician. While in high school he is advised to emphasize the biological sciences in his high school curriculum, even though the social sciences may be far more relevant. It is emphasized to the high school student that he must get good grades and a good recommendation from his teachers in order to get into a quality undergraduate college. And the situation repeats itself when going from medical school to internship to residency, from residency to hospital appointment. Every advance is both a warning and a potential roadblock. The student at all levels must adhere to his superior's expectations and whims. Such enforced conformity allows the medical profession to maintain the appearance, and it's often more than an appearance, of a solid front, from top to bottom. Even as recently as 1969, deans at Columbia University's medical school were urging their students not to grow mustaches for fear they would interfere with the doctor-patient relationship. One study of medical students showed that the choice of whether or not to wear bow ties was determined by what their superior was wearing and thought fashionable.

Yet long and rigorous training is not necessary. The MD can be well trained in five to six years. His basic skills needed for physical examination, history taking, and treatment can be acquired in a six- to twelve-week period. Long years of training with expensive tuition mean that only the relatively rich, white-skinned, conservative can afford and endure such a program. Thus the profession, which not only gives service to, but is made up primarily of, the relatively wealthy, white, conservative families, perpetuates itself in its selection process. Medical educators now speak of medical students as a "highly selected breed"; only the relatively rich can afford the expensive tuition. The AMA has, of course, until very recently fought any government support for medical school tuition. Inbreeding is encouraged. Fifty per cent of all medical students have a relative who is an MD. Such families have not only the proper funds to finance medical education, but the proper "values"—politics, religion, and race. Such families are also more likely to have the proper connections to insure admission to a college, medical school, or hospital staff. Each preceding step determines a future step.

2. *Limiting the number of medical schools.* Control of the number of medical schools by the AMA has, of course, limited the number of new physicians graduating every year. The AMA has the power to deny accreditation to a new medical school, without which that new school may not receive desperately needed federal and state funds. Thus, not only are we drastically short of manpower, but training institutions which supply our manpower are in very serious financial trouble; at least a dozen or more are so seriously underfinanced and underequipped that their standards are "only minimal." These financial difficulties are exacerbated by AMA opposition to any serious federal funding, whether for medical school construction, for tuition supplements, or for student loans.

Graduate schools other than medical schools have their students subsidized not only with free tuition but with stipends for living, making these professional areas considerably more attractive, as well as less authoritarian. When a medical resi-

dent finishes his training, he is often deeply in debt—not so
the graduate student. It's extremely difficult financially for
the medical student or intern to rear a family. This adds to
his emotional, and thus his professional, dependency on his
training institution, and he finds himself fully absorbing its
ideology and ethics. But such is not the case in other professional training schools. The PhD finishes three or four years
after undergraduate school. The MD must attend institutional training for eight years following college, and then
wait for a number of years until his medical practice reaches
the profitable level. The length of the MD's training means
he must make up a considerable deficit. The graduate student, on the other hand, immediately begins his working life
with living wages.

Graduate students have less authoritarian, less structured,
less time-consuming programs and can often readily supplement their income. The education of the MD is so authoritarian, so structured, so exhausting that no time is left for
income supplementation. Clearly, in any new comprehensive
health plan, no potential physician should be excluded from
medical school on the basis of lack of family income. There
should be no impediments to medical school admission, other
than the criterion of dedication to service.

What is particularly ironic about the AMA's opposition to
direct, public tuition supplementation is that virtually all
tuition and training is already publicly subsidized, though
indirectly. For example, public money to a medical school to
do a particular piece of research will also allow the medical
school to pay the researcher's salary not only for research, but
for teaching. His laboratory might also be used for medical
student training. All federal research grants automatically
provide for 25 to 33 per cent overhead expenses to the spon-

soring university medical center, which uses it to supplement the income it receives from tuitions. Tuitions are, therefore, publically subsidized to some extent already.

But it's basically the wealthier students who are receiving the benefits of that subsidy, as tuition at most schools still runs from $1200 to $3000 per year, thereby eliminating the poor and a large percentage of middle-class students. Again, the greatest percentage of public money, rather than serving the public, serves the privileged few. These same people who are receiving these massive public subsidies complain when someone suggests that the subsidies be extended to allow middle-class and poor students to attend medical school. At that point the cry of government intervention and control is heard; a fear of lowering standards and of "socialized medicine" is voiced.

For the profession to admit that its training and service programs are in need of federal subsidy is to admit or suggest some inadequacy in the profession's planning and expertise, as the profession has always contended that such subsidies were unnecessary. Thus, as the manpower and facility shortage goes beyond the crisis stage, more and more embarrassment is faced by the profession. In many ways the profession is correct to fear that federal subsidy may lead to federal control; but this control is more frequently being diverted to the medical-industrial complex, which increasingly plays roles the government might ordinarily play. For example, supervision and payment of medicaid and medicare administration has been in the hands of Blue Cross/Blue Shield and this supervision and administration is paid for by the government. Unfortunately the "Blues" are controlled by and accountable only to the medical-industrial complex.

Every MD who graduates has had his tuition and training

subsidized to some degree by public money—in all likelihood
close to 50 to 90 per cent of his training and tuition costs are
publicly funded in spite of AMA opposition to this inadequate and maldistributed subsidy. But in no way does the
publicly trained (i.e., at public expense) physician pay his
debt back to the public. He sets his practice up in the most
lucrative areas, to serve the richest and fewest numbers of
patients possible. Public subsidies have subsidized the increase in the disparity in the quality of care between the rich
and the poor, rather than narrowing it. Public subsidies have
subsidized a highly fragmented, multiclass, continuously inflationary health system—benefiting the privileged few and
not the public at large.

3. *Over emphasis on reading and verbal skills.* Medical
school admission aptitude tests discriminate against those
with poor literary and verbal communication skills. Such admission tests obviously discriminate economically and ra-
cially. However, no physician or potential physician has ever
been excluded because he couldn't communicate well with
blacks or Puerto Ricans or poor people, but plenty of blacks,
Puetro Ricans, and poor people have been excluded from
medical school because they achieved only average scores on
medical college admission tests. There can be alternatives to
such admission tests. Prospective medical students might be
given a three-month clinical/academic apprenticeship, during which time their potential for being physicians would be
determined. Any person showing interest, dedication, and
ability would be accepted on the basis of such attributes
rather than on the basis of their verbal cleverness. Admission
would be on the basis of dedication to service to the community and not commitment to corporate or class interests.
Optimally, there should be enough health institutions to pro-

vide openings for all who wished to serve, wherever their interests lay and in whatever capacity they were most capable.

Admission tests to college and medical schools are overloaded with upper-middle-class values and skills, which have little relevance to providing quality care. The formidable education and selection criteria clearly are geared to cut down the number of potential doctors and have been successful in this endeavor beyond the wildest dreams of the profession. But they also have created a nightmare situation where not only are we vastly undermanned, not only is the quantity of physicians kept low, but the quality of students has declined in response to a number of factors, including increasing prestige in other professions where less time, less cost, and less regimentation in training exists.

Admission to medical schools is almost totally arbitrary and often depends on the interviewer's opinion of your "personality and character." Will the prospective student tolerate hierarchies well? These are, obviously, qualifications not subject to objective measurement and leave considerable latitude for the operation of prejudice against applicants whose sex, race, and creed differ from those of the examiners.

In fact there is no way to predict quality performance in a future MD by his college grades or admission tests. Quality performance as a physician requires relatively limited technology. That is, the day-to-day care of physicians is not the heroics of open-heart surgery, but the diagnosis and treatment of the pneumonias, VD's, appendectomies, et al. (This will be more fully discussed in the section on technology.) Quality performance depends much more on his (her) humanity and concern for and interest in his (her) patients, intellectual curiosity, and a desire to serve as an equal in a partnership-for-health relationship. All these issues are much more important than grades, and despite what medical school admissions people may think, can never be determined by grades and admission tests. Thus, as one medical educator, Frank Rosenthal, noted: ". . . medicine is the only profession where the element of competition comes only at the beginning"; but even much of that competition is elminated by classism, racism, and sexism.

In getting into medical school, competition is used to protect the profession and not the patient. Quality practice comes more from caring than knowing. Economic imperatives tend more toward assembly-line practice, with little time for care or concern. Care and concern cannot be measured by grades. The use of grades and admission tests emphasizes the screen of technology, i.e., that a myth is advanced that it's important to possess an unlimited amount of technology and that you must be unlimitedly brilliant to understand, master, and use it, and that only MD's with good grades are capable of providing quality care.

4. *Discrimination against women.* The very use of the term "laity" to describe the general public underlies the profession's view of itself as a male-dominated religious order. However, professional "integrity and ethics" did not spring from religious roots, but from economic roots. Religion might be used to rationalize and legitimize them once they were in effect, but it didn't create them—the economic needs of the profession did. What sprang from the church was the economic similarity of church and profession in their emphasis on mysticism, professionalism, hierarchy, elitist selectivity, and male chauvinism. The economics of medical education is the economics of exclusion along not only racial, but sexual lines as well. Only 8 per cent of all physicians are women, in spite of the fact that they are 51 per cent of the population.

It's clear that for a woman to be admitted to medical school she needs higher grades and better recommendations than males. Thus women medical students tend to rank academically higher than their male classmates. Medical school deans often use as their rationalization for discrimination against females the fact that the women may get pregnant and then would have to devote more time to child rearing than to medical learning. Such would not be the case, of course, if day care centers were provided.

In spite of gross shortages of physicians, the medical profession has made no serious attempt to transfer skills to non-physicians, particularly females such as nurses and aides. Transfer of skills to solve manpower problems might mean a loss of money to the MD. The ophthalmologist who gets $30 per eye refraction can't get the same $30 if his nurse does it, even though she may be equally as capable, with some simple training. An extreme example of failure to transfer skills was the decade's long debate at the turn of the century over whether or not nurses should be allowed to take temperatures. It was (and all too often is) felt that women aren't emotionally stable, intellectually capable, or fit to assume such crushing responsibilities. Thus the role of women in medicine has been that of handmaiden to, and a sexual object for, the physician, there to do his bidding and bedding. Women's role in medicine is no different from their role in society in general—on the bottom.

In those areas of health care where man- and woman-power shortages have now made it an absolute necessity for nurses and other female health professionals and workers to acquire and use more skills and assume more responsibility, a concomitant shift in authority, compensation, and prestige has not followed. If a more appropriate transfer of skills to nurses and others occurred, medical students would spend more professional and training time with nurses in order to learn from them. But of course by staying away from nurses, it is easier to maintain an elitist, superior role. Nurses often must assume the front-line, hour by hour care for the patient, bail out negligent or inadequately supervised interns and residents, and yet receive little in the way of public acknowledgement or direct compensation for this.

The medical student's first educational experience is with the cadaver—the natural beginning of the death profession. Why shouldn't the first experience be with a healthy family, to understand what makes them healthy, rather than what kills them? The model for medical education should be illness prevention and health enhancement. The students' training should emphasize preventive medicine issues, e.g., vaccination, nutrition, abortion, contraception, maternal and child care. It's no coincidence that the above mentioned preventive modalities deal primarily with women and in general are neglected by the male-dominated profession, except when patients are from white, upper-middle classes.

Women, as patients, are uniquely oppressed in both the male-dominated medical and economic systems. This is so not only because men discriminate against women and objectify them, but also because women have a greater physiological need for health services than men (e.g., prenatal and postnatal care) and thus are more dependent on it.

Women make 25 per cent more visits to health facilities, and use 50 per cent more prescription drugs than men. Women suffer not only as health consumers but as health workers: 70 per cent of all health workers are women, yet they occupy the lowest-paying positions. While the health system is inadequate generally, it's specifically inadequate for women who are involved with it more than men.

In the medical system men are the decision makers, women are what the decisions are about. Men see women as passive, dependent, and irrational, and treat them as such. Commonly, pregnancy is treated as a somewhat humorous situation. As Robb Burlege of the Health Policy Advisory Center points out: "Women of almost all classes, almost uniformly hate or fear the gynecologist. He plays a controlling role in that aspect of their lives that a male-dominated society values most —the sexual aspect—and he knows it. Middle class women find a physician to be either patronizing, over-jolly, or cold and condescending. Poorer women using clinics are more likely to encounter outright brutality and sadism."

Drug companies use women as objects. In advertisements drugs are promoted by being placed adjacent to scantily clad and sexually promising women. To compound the problem of sexism in advertising is the fact that the drug may be prescribed by doctors more on the basis of its sexual appeal than on the basis of its therapeutic efficacy. More drugs are not only prescribed for women, but also more drugs are tested on women. Thus women serve as research objects, where they risk their lives; women serve to promote and advertise the same drug, and more often than not are forced to buy it on the advice of and prescription from a male doctor.

Doctors have a responsibility to their patients for providing sex education. However, very little of it occurs. The reason there has been so little of it, aside from the fact that doctors are more up tight about sex than most people, falls into three areas, all of which have an economic basis:

A. Doctors, as virtually the most privileged class or sector in America, speak most strongly for the status quo, including status-quo morals. Real sex education would involve questioning these morals and the status quo that upholds them.

B. More importantly, however, is the role of sex education, or indeed any public health or medical education the patient might receive. It tends to demystify the professional role; it transfers information to the patient and allows him to be more independent. Sex education allows the patient to get to know the physician better personally and thus is deprofessionalizing.

C. Finally, and most importantly, there is simply no profit for physicians in sex education. It's time consuming for doctors to discuss with a patient sex or anything else—and time is money. What sex education does occur, is substantively male chauvinistic. For example, the male physician will advise his young male patients that sex is "O.K." and that it's fine "to sow a few wild seeds." The physician will then discuss adequate means of contraception. For his young female patients, on the other hand, sex outside of marriage is taboo. Often the physician will not only refuse to discuss contraceptives, but worse, won't provide the means for the women to obtain them. And of course, once the woman is pregnant, he will oppose abortion.

The doctor's training and attitude about abortion are stated in the key reference, *Obstetrics,* by Eastman and Hellman who, in 1966, wrote that ". . . medical ethics do not permit abortion for sociological reasons." In a male-dominated health system, men have control over a woman's body and thus have opposed abortion on demand unless the woman was white and wealthy. Legal strictures preventing that demand from being met encouraged illegal structures to meet it. Thus, the abortion industry "is the Mafia's third most lucrative racket," says Rachel Fruchter of the New York

City Women's Abortion Project. Doctors at training centers in our university medical centers have opposed abortion because it is not an adequate training procedure for young doctors, since it is one that is boring and relatively simple.

Sexism is as American as apple pie and racism. However, the sexual "minority" of women is really a majority of 51 per cent of the population. Sexism cannot be taken out of the health system without taking it out of society and all its institutions, from the family to the medical-industrial complex.

5. *Greater use of technology.* As the economy has evolved to more complex levels, new technologies have been implemented. A greater dependency on technology and the economic impetus for its development have exacerbated seriously the manpower problem. For more and more technology, more and more researchers and technicians are needed to design and develop it; more and more research programs and patients are needed to refine it—thus fragmenting care. The more technology available, the more rationalizations are given for the need for longer periods of training for all health workers, thus again intensifying the manpower problem, extending the hierarchies, increasing mystique and professionalism, and inflating the cost of health care. The longer the training program, the less attractive and the more exclusionary the profession. The future MD—the medical student—is forced to master a lot of irrelevant facts about technology, irrelevant to quality care, but not irrelevant to the medical economic structure. The most important part of conventional health care is not lab equipment or technology, but a time-consuming medical history and physical examination. The current medical system, however, encourages cursory examinations and symptomatic treatment.

The possession or existence of technology has little or no

connection with whether or not it will be used or used properly. For example, in Osler Petersen's famous study of general practitioners, 43 per cent of the GP's were observed
using improperly sterilized instruments. What's missing is not
technology, but concern for the patient. But such concern is
not part of medical education or the medical system.

At a different level, being receptive to technological inno-
vation has nothing to do with working for the implementation of those innovations or at least not opposing them, as
the profession has frequently done.

6. *Unnecessary procedures and operations.* A number of
studies have shown that at least a hundred thousand hysterectomies are done unnecessarily each year. There are also thousands of unnecessary tonsillectomies performed each year.
Both operations are indicative of our illness-for-profit system.
Not only are unnecessary operations dangerous (about ten
thousand deaths occur every year just from the anesthesia
connected to the surgical procedure), they also inflate the
price of health care and are an unnecessary drain on manpower and facilities.

Other factors play a role in exacerbating the manpower
problems but are not necessarily caused or promoted by the
profession. For instance, a recent cause for the decrease in the
number of medical school applicants is the increasing integration, coordination, and bureaucratization of medical practice. It's increasingly more difficult to be a rugged individ-
ualist and one man entrepreneur in contemporary medical
practice. At the very minimum you need hospital admitting
privileges, ancillary help, especially in dealing with the de-
luge of insurance forms and processes, both private and public. Medical practice and the doctor are increasingly just a
cog in the wheel of a large corporate enterprise. This turns

away from the medical arena some potential physicians, who do not wish to be lost in a bureaucratization process. This decline in number and quality of physicians is particularly alarming in view of the fact that we're entering a period—with no end in sight—of greater and greater need for physicians and health workers.

In spite of the profession's vocal support for the free enterprise system, they have failed to abide by one of its basic tenets: "that the recruited supply be equated with the manifested demand." Supply has never matched demand and has been farther away than ever from meeting needs. The free market the profession speaks of is the freedom to limit competition and engage in price gouging.

An increase in the flow of new medical recruits poses not only the threat of greater competition but also the risk of bringing in people who differ substantially from those already there: more blacks, browns, women, homosexuals, and poorer people—all of whom may have a different political orientation and sense of public service than have the existing professionals. In a truly free and truly competitive market, different ideas and systems are allowed to compete with one another. For example, medical school training, as currently carried on, is probably not the cheapest, most efficient, quickest way to train MD's. Open-ended career ladder programs, avoiding much of college and book-type education, and instead substituting experience and on-the-job training and apprenticeship, might train surgeons much more quickly and more effectively than the current methods.

As a monopoly, the medical profession is all too likely to confuse its own interest with the public interest. By having monopoly powers over the medical market place, the profession has been able to resort to exploitive methods to limit some of the grosser aspects of manpower shortages. Some of these exploitive methods are:

1. *Foreign trained physicians.* As I have said . . . in an attempt to limit competition, the AMA has worked to limit the number of practicing physicians by limiting medical school admissions and controlling licensing. However, the profession has created such a monstrous shortage of physicians that it must compensate for this. Thus county medical societies have been allowing poorly trained foreign physicians to work in hospitals as interns and residents, so that American physicians can avoid emergency and night duties. Twenty-five to thirty per cent of all interns and residents are now foreign trained. The foreign trained professionals are thus a source of cheap labor brought here to relieve the American physician. These imported physicians readily submit to professional authority, as the threat of loss of a visa can be particularly intimidating. Professional control of licensing, specialty boards, and hospital accreditation boards allows for easy importation and channeling of foreign physicians to maintain our multiclass health delivery system. The influx of foreign-trained physicians has been just enough to stave off federal intervention to solve physician manpower problems. Not only does the importation of foreign professionals allow this country to avoid solving its manpower problems, it also creates and exacerbates professional manpower problems in countries which are desperately poor and export their physicians to the United States. India, with a population over twice that of ours, with half as many physicians, sends each year to this country scores of doctors. The number of physicians we import each year is about the same as we graduate from our own medical schools. The cost to build and maintain our medical educational institutions runs in the neighborhood of $10 bil-

lion a year, which in effect we extract from poorer countries when we import their physicians in numbers equivalent to the numbers we graduate. Even worse than the economic loss to these countries is the loss in lives caused by their physician shortage. The "brain drain" of, say, physicians coming to the United States from India is catastrophic to the fragile Indian health system.

Because foreign physicians in this country represent a potential source of competition, it is extremely difficult for them to get permanent licenses to go into private practice. Thus, foreign MD's can practice, in general, only as interns and residents, where they are poorly paid and where they treat patients with whom they often cannot communicate because of language barriers. The language barrier alone can become a danger to human life. The only opening in American medical practice for these foreigners is usually in the GP area in the central city, rapidly being vacated for the suburbs and the more lucrative specialties. These foreign physicians go into general practice because there are fewer roadblocks to general practice. They thus practice in the ghetto or rural areas where they will be the least supervised/ or observed, or both, by any medical society or evaluatory organization. They are forced to practice where the profits are lowest, but the people the sickest, and they, as foreign physicians, the least equipped to handle that degree of sickness. Therefore the importation of foreign trained MD's has a doubly racist nature:

A. They come from countries where nonwhites predominate, e.g., India, Korea, Phillipines, and so on, and deprive those nonwhite countries of physicians.

B. They practice often predominantly in our black, brown, and yellow ghettos, where the profession and MIC have perpetrated a chronic inadequacy in health care. The foreign physician in the ghetto more often than not has an inadequate hospital backup.

2. *Utilization of foreign medical schools as educational resources for training American doctors.* With the tremendous shortage of MD's in this country created by the purposefully created shortage of medical schools, numerous United States citizens and potential physicians seek training in foreign medical schools, depriving that country of its own limited resources (a place in a medical school and a potential future doctor) to increase our own. However, we are somewhat saved the economic embarrassment of having to deal with these manpower issues. The profession does not have to worry about federal intervention in medical training if manpower deficits can be somewhat minimized by using training facilities in other countries. Of course the United States physicians trained in most foreign medical schools are not as adequately prepared as they could be if they went to American schools. In comparison, Russia has a sufficient supply of MD's available to lend to poorer countries from whom we take. Russia has almost 200 doctors for every 100,000 persons; we have only 135. Clearly their priorities are different from ours, and ours won't be changed by any of the proposed new health legislation.

3. *Charity patients for research and training.* Manpower shortages create a multiclass system of health care, insuring wide areas of medical indigency.

The character of training, function, and practice has been professionally determined to be along lines of illness removal and not health enhancement. Since illness can be used as a marketable commodity and health cannot, there is an investment in illness. Since we live in a class and class-exploitive society, there is a maximal investment in illness in the lowest classes. Thus we see the development of a multiclass system of health care where the poor are used as training cases by students, interns, and residents, in order that they may be competent by the time they go into practice in comparatively wealthier neighborhoods. Again, mirroring the economic system, the blacks and Puerto Ricans, who are most excluded from the benefits of the economic system, are the people not only most excluded from the benefits of the health system but also the people most exploited by it. Those most exploited by, and most deprived of, the benefits of the health system are often the fatal victims of that system, that is, they die as a result of that system. These deaths are a constant reminder of the violence perpetrated by both the economic and health systems. These deaths are the reason why organizations such as the Medical Liberation Front have called the American Medical Association the "American Murder Association." Poor people and the medically indigent pay for their medical bills with their bodies. These bodies are used for the testing of new, untried medicines, often without the legally required informed consent of the patient. The body of the medically indigent is essentially raw material to be exploited. Drug experimentation brings in money from the drug companies and federal granting agencies. The drugs are first tried on the poor, and if proved to be efficacious are then purchased by the nonmedically indigent. The poor, invariably, without private physicians, rarely get to utilize the results of the research until it is too late and they are dying in the hospital.

University medical centers train their medical students by giving them considerable, though often illegitimate, responsibility for the care of indigent patients. It is with these patients that medical students are to learn by their mistakes, so they won't make them when they go to the suburbs, but rather will be self-reliant. The patient as raw material is nothing but a training device. Nurses often have to bail out the medical students covering for them and correcting their mistakes. The student also learns how to lie and deceive patients about his own ambivalence and lack of skills, thus dehumanizing his patients as well as himself. Those patients who aren't utilizable as teaching and research material are sent to the nearest municipal hospital ("the dumping syndrome").

Much of medical training is an apprenticeship, observing the examples set by one's superior and absorbing their values. The examples set, however, are neglect and poor care for the poor patient. Medical instructors are more interested in their private research projects or private practices, leaving the medical student free to order and prescribe unnecessary and often dangerous drugs and tests. After all, the poor patient is there to serve the university medical center and not the other way around.

Patients are publicly embarrassed for teaching purposes. In one particular case when a young female patient was disrobed to her waist before 130 male medical students, the teacher seemed to think that the patient was unduly embarrassed—"after all, they're just medical students here to learn something." The teacher thought the patient's anxiety was symptomatic of neurosis. When the medical students paraded by the girl to examine her, one by one, which included feeling her breasts, she of course became more anxious, which the teacher again dismissed as a neurotic symptom of coquettishness. Numerous unnecessary exams and procedures are a part of the everyday life of the charity patient.

4. *Use of medical students and house staff as cheap sources*

of labor. Long years of training, financial and emotional dependency on the profession and its institutions, and an authoritarian system producing submissiveness, allow medical students and house staff to be used as cheap labor. Under the guise of being educated during an apprenticeship, i.e., the clinical years of medical school, internship, and residency, the student, intern, or resident is paid little or nothing but given a considerable part of the work load, relieving the supervising physicians not only from many aspects of patient care, but also from their teaching responsibilities. "Scut" work (i.e., dirty work) is foisted upon the student in the name of medical education.

Students, interns, and residents are a cheap source of labor, supposedly in exchange for the education they are receiving, though actually most of the education students, interns, and residents receive is not from their supervising physicians or conferences but from their own trial and error—experimentation—the practice of medicine on willing and unknowing charity patients, unfortunate enough to be sick in a teaching ward. By extending the time spent in training, you extend the time spent in servitude. Each step ahead depends on the step before. No wonder medical students are so intimidated by the time they complete their residency. They must behave and conform in college and get good grades to go to medical school. The behaving and conformity is then repeated each year in medical school and then cumulatively for internship and then for residency and then for post—residency hospital appointment. The process is indoctrination ideologically and not medically.

One does not need to be a physician or some technical expert to know that we are drastically short of health professionals. Thus the decision to deal with the problem as effectively and efficiently, by whatever means necessary, should not be left in the hands of the profession that created the problem in the first place.

The medical profession, recognizing tremendous manpower shortages at last (a recognition forced on them by threats from the government) can move in a number of ways:

Either the profession can train more physicians or transfer more skills to nonphysicians. The profession would like to do neither of these. To train more physicians ultimately involves increased public subsidies with the potential for public control of the profession. More physicians means increasing competition among physicians. To transfer skills to nonphysicians means some degree of deprofessionalization, demystification, and with it, the possible necessity to transfer not only skills, but power, privilege, prestige, and profit. Notice how the profession's "problems" are really solutions for the people.

The profession seems to be opting for training a few more MD's and using federal money to do so with the hope that even if "worst came to worst" the government would control only medical education and not medical practice. Probably at the same time is the recognition that even if we increase by 50 per cent the existing number of university medical centers, an extremely unlikely event at present, given the cost of almost $100 million per new quality university medical center, there would be only an additional three to four thousand more MD's a year, which is only 1 to 2 per cent of the present total. Thus 1 to 2 per cent more MD's a year won't seriously improve the manpower problem or bring better health care, which is precisely why the profession is opting for this "solution"—because it really isn't a solution.

On the other hand, increasing the time effectiveness of our

300,000 MD's by transferring skills to others, for example, physical exams (all or part), suturing and other procedures, and by saving the MD only 5 per cent of his time, would be the equivalent of almost 15,000 new MD's. This real solution becomes even more necessary when we realize the trend toward specialization is only about midway complete. As it becomes more complete, the manpower problem will worsen further. At least 50 per cent of new specialists are really subspecialists. That is, no one simply specializes in surgery, they subspecialize in orthopedic surgery or hand surgery or pediatric surgery, and so on. Psychiatrists are increasingly limiting their practice to child psychiatry, or community psychiatry, or group psychiatry. While there are some programs extant and proposed for transfer of medical skills, they are few in number and only at an experimental level. Professional control of licensing regulations, for one, limits the general implementation of transference of skills. The physician shortage leaving the patient no choice of physician allows the MD to charge virtually as he sees fit.

While it is true that MD's fees are a major factor in the inflationary price rise, the evil of the system isn't the level of their incomes as much as it is the way in which fees render medical care inaccessible. Over all the problem, in terms of physicians' fees, is that there are at present no mechanisms to control fees. The profession has a monopoly on the market and they can charge whatever the traffic will bear. Even agencies such as Blue Cross and Blue Shield, which are supposed to insure that the public are charged only "reasonable" fees, have on their boards of directors people who are more responsive to doctors and the medical-industrial complex than to the patient-consumer. And where fees are held down, i.e., where the Blue Cross-Blue Shield doesn't reimburse the

MD or hospital the full amount billed for, he or the hospital simply charges the remainder to the patient.

Because of monopoly control and physician shortages, physicians go where the money is, that is, where the market is profitable and not where it is poor. The distribution of physicians, rather than being based on need, is located precisely along income lines, where the need is least. Since the poorest patients are also the sickest and the sickest the poorest, the poor areas have the greatest health needs, but it's here that there is the lowest distribution of MD's, nurses, facilities, and so forth, and what facilities there are, are second rate. For example, Bellevue Hospital in New York City, the major charity hospital in Manhattan, has to be excused year after year for not meeting accreditation standards, in spite of the fact that it's supposed to serve one of the largest patient populations in the world.

The maximum supply of physicians is thus in the suburbs and in practices affiliated with prestigious university and voluntary medical centers. The supply is lowest in ghetto and rural areas. Thus, in spite of the fact that all medical schools are publicly financed for the majority of their funds, physicians are trained to treat the upper classes by first practicing on, learning from, and exploiting the poorer classes. The relevance of the above to the manpower issue is that New Deal type legislation, that is, the pouring of more and more money into a rotten system to solve manpower problems, only serves to perpetuate that system without even solving the manpower problem. The federal influx of money into the health educational system has increased the disparity between the care the upper classes receive and that which the lower classes receive.

Manpower shortages leave the physician with the choice of

doing a proper job for some patients while neglecting the others, or doing an inadequate job for larger numbers of patients. Thus the concept of health care as a right is impossible under the present system of manpower inadequacies. Even if the medically indigent were suddenly given the money to purchase care, there wouldn't be enough physicians to dispense it, nor would they be evenly distributed enough to be located and accessible.

Specialization

Analagous to the old-time general store is the general practitioner or family physician. The GP is rapidly becoming less important, at least numerically, in the health arena. Recent polls of graduating medical school classes show that less than 5 per cent of the senior class members plan to become GP's. The drop in the number of general practitioners mirrors the decline and fall of AMA membership and influence. The AMA since its inception has been made up of, and controlled by, the general practitioner—the individual entrepreneur of the health arena.

The American Medical Association has undergone within the last five to ten years a considerable decline in membership, to the point where they represent only 50.6 per cent of licensed MD's in the country. By the end of 1971 they will no longer represent a majority of United States physicians.

Where have all the GP's gone? A number of factors have led to their declining influence, such as advances in technology, evolving institutional and bureaucratic imperatives, and most importantly, the sway of monopoly economics.

In an attempt to maximize profits, attempts to gain monopolistic control over parts of the body were initiated. Thus, general practitioners battle specialists, various types of specialists battle one another, as each is engaged in an imperialistic struggle to expand its domain over segments of the human anatomy. As Adam Smith noted almost two hundred years ago in his *Wealth of Nations*, the extent of specialization tends to vary with the extent and advancement of the economy.

Professor Elton Raycock, of the University of Rhode Island, medical economist wrote in 1967: "Fundamentally, what is involved here is exactly the same kind of social conflict generated by the internal contradiction inherent in the concept of professionalism. Society has given organized medicine the power to set quality standards in order to protect the patient. But organized medicine has frequently used that power as a restrictionist device with socially undesirable results, e.g., manpower shortages and fragmented care, in order to increase the incomes, power, and prestige of its members. In a sense, ironically, the general practitioners are caught in a trap largely of their own making. They have always been, as have physicians generally, vigorous proponents of the policy that only medical doctors have the right to set standards for medical practice; only then, they argued, would adequate quality standards be maintained to protect the patient. And it is precisely this kind of argument that the specialists have used against the general practitioners." In effect specialists are saying that only if the various kinds of practice are restricted to the appropriate specialist, only if the various specialty boards and specialty board members set standards in and out of hospitals, can adequate quality be maintained. Thus we see the power of specialty training as a tool for monopolistic and exclusionary control over parts of the body. As GP's battle specialists and specialists battle each other, organized medicine is faced with a dilemma similar to that which bedevils society in its relationship with organized medicine as a whole: When does the power to set quality standards, a power too often considered socially desirable to delegate to professionals, become a device for restricting practice with socially undesirable results?

Another means of limiting competition is limiting the numbers and types of physicians who get hospital staff privileges. As Dr. Raycock points out: "Without hospital staff privileges, or with privileges severely limited, the physician must relinquish a patient (as well as fees) requiring hospitalization to a specialist having access to a hospital." In light of the fact that nearly half of medical incomes are now earned in hospitals, the impetus to build hospitals, to treat patients in hospitals, and to restrict doctors from hospitals must be seen in terms of its economic causation rather than simply a concern for patient welfare. The restrictions of staff privileges is thus not an attempt to raise medical standards in hospitals so much as it is a monopolistic device for limiting competition in order to protect and increase the incomes of specialists entrenched in hospital practice.

Numerous studies suggest that specialty board certification for hospital privileges is no guarantee of adequate quality and in fact suggests that restrictive measures exist more out of concern for eliminating competition than for insuring quality.

Increased specialization has led to increased fragmentation of health services. The increase in specialists means longer training periods and thus delays before full services can be given. The great percentage rise in specialists and the concommitant percentage decline in GP's mean patients enter the health system increasingly by first seeing a specialist—

often the wrong kind—who in turn must refer the patient to the appropriate specialist. This is fine for the specialists involved in the referring system, but it is time consuming and costly for the patient while he finds the appropriate specialist. It means that the initial referring specialist was expensively overtrained if he serves only to refer the patient. The above suggests how care is fragmented, the cost inflated, profits maximized by multiple referrals, and the patient made increasingly dependent, confused, and financially drained.

A Harvard surgeon, Dr. Francis Moore, said about the irrationality of specialty training: ". . . I never understood why certain specialty boards permitted one to become a specialist and operate on certain organs of the body after 2 years, while other specialty boards required 5 years of residency before one was permitted to operate on other organs." Dr. E. Ginzburg at Columbia University follows up: "It should be clear, that we cannot indefinitely extend the period of medical and specialty training on the assumption that the more the better. In this connection it is well to recall . . . that an average fully fledged member of the American Psychoanalytic Association did not complete all of his training until after his fortieth year. Small wonder that psychoanalysts charge large fees. They have only a short time in which to recover for years of outlay."

One reason for the decline in quality and quantity of medical school applicants is the increasingly long time required to be a specialist. Some specialty residencies are now up to five and six years beyond internship. Such indentured servitude does not add to the profession's attractiveness, especially when that servitude requires working an eighty-hour week at an average of only two to three dollars an hour—and it's only

relatively recently that the compensation has been that high
—in a highly structured, authoritarian atmosphere.

Expanding knowledge and technology have been increasingly used as a rationalization to extend the length of training periods, while the real reasons reside more in the area of
preserving economic privileges and excluding competition.

As less and less GP's are trained, the patient's first contact
with the health system is often the specialists. In the ghetto
it's even worse—it's the pharmacist or the herbist; all of
which is to say that specialists are overtrained in terms of
being the initial contact, and pharmacists are undertrained.
We do need a free, readily available, competent health worker
for the purposes required for first, primary contact and referral. A specialist, given our limited resources, is both expensively overtrained and overpaid.

A specialist has been described as "a person who learns
more and more about less and less." Being insecure about
anything outside his limited orbit, he is apt to be overly sus-
picious and to order a series of expensive, and often unnecessary, tests right off the bat. "In the care of such common and
obscure complaints as persistent headaches, the patient is
likely to wind up with a neurological consultation and an
electroencephalograph and still be no better off." The specialist might also tend to refer more to other specialists than
might the GP, who might have more fear of losing a patient
to a specialist. For example, there are three different ways an
ulcer might be evaluated, diagnosed, treated, and referred.
An internist might recommend conservative medical management with drugs, a surgeon might recommend surgery, and a
psychiatrist might recommend psychotherapy. Others might
recommend a combination of the above. It is extremely hard
to know who is correct. The point to remember, however,

is that there is a motivation for maximal referral because of reciprocation for referral and fee splitting where the referring physician gets a percentage of the bill charged to his patient by the "referred to" physician, all of which fragments care and decreases accountability; all of which is extremely expensive given the great investment in the training of these specialists; none of which has anything to do with providing maximal quality.

Surgeons, at the top of the economic heap, in general have been opposed to fee splitting, but only because it cuts into their income. In spite of the fact that the AMA has called fee splitting "unethical," it has gotten around this in the surgical area by saying the GP could assist the surgeon in the operating room and be reimbursed for it. This was an attempt not only to allow fee splitting to continue, but to get the GP into the hospital from which he might ordinarily be excluded. At other times it is an ineffectual ethic for window dressing only.

Fragmentation of services, specialization, and colonization of the patient's anatomy all result in ignoring the patient as a whole and his mental and social environment, even though the mental and social context might play a greater etiological role than his physical causes and symptoms. But to look at the mental and social context is time consuming for the specialists and raises too many embarrassing questions, for example, about the narrowness of the professional definition and the quality of medical care and training. There is no profit in relating to mental and social issues, unless the physician did it in the narrow context of the specialist-psychiatrist.

Specialists can set shorter hours for themselves by being responsible for less and less. But claiming to know more and more for what they are responsible, they can charge more on a per visit basis. Specialists, because of their more years of training and an apparent greater deal of knowledge, have added to the caste system, which used to consist of MD-Nurse-Aide, and so on, and is now specialist-GP-nurse-aide, and so on. Those on top of the hierarchy are in a better position to control the financial and social arrangements of medical care, as when lack of specialization is used as an excuse to deny hospital privileges to GP's and therefore to deny them access to patients and their money.

By not allowing GP's hospital privileges, there is created a self-fulfilling prophecy: GP's are not given privileges because it is said they are not competent, and then when they are not given privileges and denied the learning atmosphere and resources of the teaching hospital, it introduces and insures their continued incompetence and ignorance.

Specialization has led to fragmentation of care. If you go to a GP who doesn't have hospital privileges and if you do need hospitalization, you will have to go to another MD who does have hospital privileges. Therefore, the GP without privileges faces the risk of losing you as a patient. Why should the patient return to the MD who doesn't have privileges? Therefore, the ethic that an MD is not supposed to "steal" patients is circumvented by those with hospital privileges, to exclude and "steal" from those without it. Specialists charge more and control more because they have greater access to and control of the wealthier population; the GP's get the poorer patients and many patients get no one. By creating a caste system, people who want the "best" turn to specialists. GP's become the untouchables. Specialization also forces MD's to distribute themselves geographically in certain ways, so that rural areas are totally devoid of specialists, as there are no hospitals and allied technology for use by the specialist. As fewer and fewer young medical students become GP's, the age of GP's increases. GP's tend to be isolated from hospitals, often out in rural areas, so that there is an increasing disparity of care between the best and the worst care—especially with the specialist monopolizing the richest clientele. Where GP's are replaced by younger GP's, the latter tend to be foreign trained. All of which is to say that health care is where the money is, not where the need is.

The incongruity of specialization is that the MD who covers the widest area of practice, the GP, receives the shortest period of preparation and continuity of training. There is possibly a real place for the GP in screening, referring, chronic management of chronic diseases, and treatment and diagnosis of some of the more common diseases, e.g., pneumonia, neuroses, and so on. But such a place has not yet been arranged on the basis of health need. The American Academy of General Practice has now attempted to make General Practice or Family Practice into a specialty. However, this attempt was at creating a new specialty, not along lines of control of an organ but along lines of control of who sees the patient first. Their attempts at specialization are as economically motivated as are the other specialties.

There is no evidence that specialization has improved the standards of medical care and enhanced its effectiveness. It has the potential for doing these things, just as new technology has potentials, but to be real, they must be implemented and accessible and not fragmented and inaccessible. Specialization has decreased continuity of care; the patient makes the rounds from one specialist to another, not one of whom assumes responsibility. Specialization often means no "unified management and responsibility" for the patient.

"Specialization is a more certain guarantee that one knows little outside his own field, than he is really expert within it." Specialization "leads to undue emphasis on isolated organic systems and excessive use of lab procedures," preoccupation with narrowly defined medical problems, and dims the view of the multiple origins frequently figuring in disease.

Specialization and hospitalization complement one another, but not to the betterment of the patient. Together both allow monopolization of the anatomy and the technology and personnel that relate to medical care and illness. Specialists, by the nature of their training and the system under which they practice, are even more disease-and-curative oriented and not prevention oriented as GP's might be. After all, the patient wouldn't be referred to a specialist for primary prevention of a disease—only the care and cure of it.

Specialty Boards' certification is a form of superspecialization. When an MD has finished his residency, he is called "board eligible" in that specialty. To narrow the competition further, MD's are asked to take additional tests, usually about two years after completion of their residency, to be considered "board certified." Many hospitals won't give out hospital admitting privileges to just board-eligible specialists; they must be board certified. Thus by the time board certification is gained, it is two years beyond the twelve years of training.

Since specialists, especially medical-center based ones, are increasingly gaining control over hospitals, and since the practice of medicine increasingly, at least on a financial level, occurs in hospitals, specialists and their certifying boards have greater control than ever of the profession. The AMA, on the other hand, which has generally been dominated by rural GP's, whose numbers in the country have been rapidly decreasing due to aging, dying off, and not being replaced, has experienced a decline in its control of the profession. Thus, there is competition within the profession itself between the specialists, their hospitals, as well as related health industries and the GP-dominated AMA, which is being more and more excluded from access to patients and technology.

Specialization, while superficially setting higher standards, has not necessarily done so. Specialization may have raised people's expectations and thus their demands, but in actuality it has fragmented services, inflated the price of them, wasted resources, and overrelied on technology.

Since getting certification takes an even longer time, it means large numbers of physicians are excluded from certification, thereby only adding to the medical hierarchy. On an economic basis, surgery, at the moment, is the most lucrative specialty. It requires the most endurance and obedience in training, the most technology, facilities, personnel, and equipment. It is the most restrictive in its membership. It attracts the most conservative people, has the tightest hierarchial arrangements and the greatest monopoly control. It has the most concern about organicity and the least for personal and social factors. It is also no coincidence that in this specialty there are more lawsuits filed, there are greater manpower shortages, the greatest abuses in terms of carelessness, and worse, unnecessary operations and thus unnecessary deaths.

The surgeon in many ways has the most organized and channelized markets. In general, only surgeons do surgery, have access to surgical patients, operating rooms, nurses, equipment and anesthesiologists. The surgeon pays nothing for his publicly bought (via the hospital) tools and equipment. Thus the surgeon adds, to his financial assets, those of the hospital. It takes an internist (a specialist in internal medicine) treating a hospitalized coronary patient, about 4 weeks of daily hospital visits to collect the equivalent of a surgeon's fee for a routine appendectomy, which along with postoperative visits usually accounts for no more than 3 or 4 hours of the surgeon's time. The mystique of death and life heroism has also enhanced the surgeon's ability to charge what the market will bear, even though the skill and judgment of the surgeon may be below that of the family doctor who made the original diagnosis.

The issue isn't whether or not there should be board certification, but that if there are such qualifying mechanisms, they be publicly accountable and used to insure quality performance and not competition limitations, mystique, and higher fees for services. If the specialty boards were really concerned about quality performance they wouldn't test the specialist just at the beginning of his career, but throughout —especially to see if he acquires new information and technology as it is developed. But even this insures very little. What one says or does before a board of examiners has nothing to do with one's practice when alone with a patient. What is needed is public scrutiny of medical records (with names of patients excluded) to insure that the MD is at least keeping up-to-date, legible, and utilizable records; that he is prescribing and referring correctly and appropriately; that he is doing the proper screening and preventive tests, e.g., Pap smears, maternal and child care programs, and so forth, and that he is submitting to pathology examination all tissues to make sure no surgery is done on normal tissues. Board certification at present is no guarantee of competence or concern.

Increased technology served to increase mystification and service expectation more than it did the need for specialists.

The fact remains that for the overwhelming number of diseases and illnesses, few specialists are needed, particularly when compared to the need for direct, primary, personal, and family services. The impetus to find new sources of money, new markets, and new customers has far more to do with expanding health technology and increasing specialization than does patient-service priorities. Thus, in consumer-controlled institutions these priorities would be reversed. There would be less emphasis on specialization and technology and more on provision of human services. Specialization is not a consequence of expanding knowledge, but of an economic evolvement to higher forms of capitalism, monopoly control, and anatomical imperialism.

While group practice entails some accountability, it is only to other MD's. GP's have a role to play in decentralized group practice which are prepaid or free services, but that doesn't mean they will be assured of an equal footing with other physician specialists. Only community control of health care can insure that and also insure a greater continuity and accountability of care because the health system is the community's and thus is made to serve the patient and not the profession.

PROFESSIONALIZATION AND DOCTOR DOMINATION

In its simplest form the medical profession is not a health profession, but an illness profession. It profits only when people are ill and never when they are well. When people are well (or *think* they are well) they don't come to the doctor's office or clinic and thus there is no profit incentive to keep patients well, only to keep them returning constantly in need of more care. The imperialization or control of the ideology defines what responsibilities and services doctors offer. These services are medical or illness services and not health or preventive services.

Accordingly, the profession will treat your lung cancer with great seriousness and admonitions about your excessive smoking, but is not about to lobby against the tobacco industry which caused the cancer in the first place. (The tobacco industry not long ago gave $10 million to the AMA "for research.") The profession is pathology and disease oriented and not health oriented. Indeed, there is almost a spectrum or continuum of illness orientation that the profession follows. For example, inpatient hospital service is preferred to outpatient service; doctor's offices are preferred over the patient's home. The greater the outreach nature of the program, the greater its preventive nature, the less likely it will win the profession's favor. Professional emphasis is on acute, short-term emergency-type treatment and not on chronic, rehabilitation services. Professional control of the ideology also allows the profession to control the technology, facilities, and personnel associated with the ideology.

The profession's maintenance of an illness ideology, or as they call it, "the medical model," allows physicians to dominate the health arena. Their rationalization goes that since health is really a problem of illness removal only physicians are qualified to do the removal of the illness. However, the United Nations' World Health Organization has sought to define health in terms other than the absence of illness. Namely, that health is a state of physical, mental, and social well-being. With this kind of ideology there would be a much greater emphasis on health and not on illness, on prevention, social and psychological issues, and not illness issues. An ideology which emphasizes health enhancement and social well-

being would sooner allow a sociologist to be the maker of
health policy than a physician—especially in view of the recognition that major improvements in health, particularly in
the health enhancement and preventive areas, have come
more from social and political changes (e.g. improvements in
housing, income, nutrition, sewage, and so forth) than from
medical technology.

In the area of psychiatry, medical or illness models are
grossly inadequate, especially when one believes that the
major causitive factors in mental "illness" are political, social,
and economic factors. This would suggest that psychiatric
problems best be dealt with by sociologists and economists,
rather than by physicians. Physicians have no training in or
understanding of broad social, political, and economic issues,
except when they relate to the profession's profits, as opposed
to the people's health. Physicians have purposefully and narrowly defined their role to deal only with the immediate illness, and not its political, social, or economic antecedents.
To deal with such issues would raise too many embarrassing
questions about the profession's collusion with numerous
disease makers, for example, lobbying with the tobacco industry, major polluters, and members of the military-industrial complex. When the issues are political or social, it's clear
that MD's are ill prepared to truly and comprehensively
serve their clients and are unlikely to, given the difficulty in
collecting a fee for such services.

Science and technology are emphasized in medical education, even though the social, psychological, and political
sciences are equally as important in the delivery of health
services. But they don't mystify, they can't be controlled,
channeled, and monopolized the way "hard" sciences and

machinery can. They also have the potential for making visible too many problems of the health system.

The facts are that medical schools have not adjusted their educational fare to meet society's changing needs and demands. Again prevention and rehabilitation are not emphasized; training programs, though there have been a few exceptions, are not geared to deal with chronic disease issues.

A *New Yorker* cartoon drawing of a very angry patient talking to a jubilant doctor is a good example of rewarding disease emphasis and ideology. The doctor says, "You only contracted the disease, Mrs. Harris. I discovered it, so it's going to be named after me." Not only is this a good example of white-coat privileges, but it demonstrates how medical training and practice emphasize disease and pathology and not health and well-being. There are no rewards for the MD who keeps his patients healthy.

The only time a physician will work in a preventive-medicine program is when he is well paid to do so, as in industrial health screening programs. In this case medicine is used as a tool for labor maintenance, in order to insure the continuity of maximum worker productivity and management profits for major corporations.

Preventive techniques, such as mass screening and early detection, are technically simple, which is precisely why the profession is uninterested in them. They not only often prevent illness, they also offer little opportunity for the building of professional mystique, control, and profit. Or worse, mass screenings might make visible some professionally embarrassing results, for example, that we are not the healthiest nation in the world—indeed, far from it. Mass screenings undoubtedly would uncover a lot of disease, raising questions about physicians who failed to diagnose them or look for them, or

the general inaccessibility of quality health care. Newly uncovered diseases would place tremendous burdens on our already short supply of health personnel, forcing the federal
government to intervene more drastically than the profession
might prefer.

Mass screening might raise difficult questions in another
area. For example, what little lead-poison screening has been
done in New York City has suggested that upwards of a hundred thousand children suffer from it, with symptoms ranging
all the way from irritability and lethargy to mental retarda-
tion and coma. The ultimate treatment, of course, is prevention. To prevent lead poisoning would mean clearing the
walls of almost one million substandard dwellings in New
York City. This of course would require a tremendous political confrontation with the powerful real-estate interests of
the city, which the medical profession, or indeed anyone else,
is unlikely to undertake. The city's response is to hide all its
lead-screening kits, to remove the issue from public scrutiny
and thus from solution. Only after numerous sit-ins in the
City's Department of Health did the Health Commissioner
make available some lead-testing kits.

The mass-screening issue is being somewhat modified by
the evolving and emerging power of the medical-industrial
complex—a power often in opposition to the profession. In
this case a number of major corporations are developing
mass-screening devices and wish to market them. Of course
they will be of no value if there are no, or inadequate, or inaccessible services to deal with the diseases uncovered.

Preventive services, such as vaccination, are literally one-
shot affairs, where only one fee is paid. The nurse's handling
of this procedure does not enhance the physician's prestige, nor
does the single visit improve his pocketbook. Thus, when med-

ical technology was advanced in this case, that is, the development of vaccinations, the profession opposed it, as they have the implementation of numerous other preventive-oriented medical advances. Professional profits are in illness, not its prevention. There's no profit in air-pollution prevention, but there is in the emphysema, bronchitis, and heart disease caused by the pollution. Control of air pollution also would not require a physician's services, but an engineer's. Thus, there is an implied vested interest in the continuation of air pollution, or at least little incentive in its removal.

The AMA has opposed Blue Cross, Social Security, free inoculation for diptheria, smallpox, and polio, VD clinics, Red Cross bloodbanks, group practice, and federal grants for mothers and children's programs.

They also opposed the elimination of means test for crippled children. The means test proved that patients couldn't afford a physician and therefore the physician didn't want and wasn't interested in that patient. The means test therefore took any ethical, moral, or financial obligations off the MD. The purpose of any means test is to separate the "good," that is, the paying customers from the "bad," that is, the poor. Because of such opposition to any health reform I once called the AMA "the American Murder Association." However, since they didn't intentionally plan on all the deaths that resulted from their opposition to such programs, to be more precise one should call them the "American Manslaughter Association."

Social reforms such as in the area of sanitation have wiped out a good deal of acute infectious emergencies as well as other acute emergencies. Thus, the greatest single health care issue today, at least numerically, is the management of chronic diseases. However, medical school training is for the acute type care and not for chronic management and rehabilitation. There's very little heroism, mystique, or money in managing the problems of old age. As the Dean of Mount Sinai School of Medicine said: "The emphasis in dealing with the prevailing disorders of middle and old age must be on the basis of preventative therapy and early diagnosis, maintenance rather than care, rehabilitation of the handicapped and much more attention to the emotional and social aspects of illness. These are precisely the areas that our existing organization of medical services is least equipped to handle adequately, with the result that many urgent needs are either wholly neglected or only partially met."

MD's don't like to work with chronic diseases. Aside from the depressing aspects of it, the elderly are among the poorest and sickest segments of our population and thus need the most care and offer the MD the least remuneration—which is precisely why chronic-disease management is avoided as an educational issue in medical school. The passage of Medicaid might change that somewhat as it might stabilize the market for management of chronic disease. The chronicity of the disease makes the patients "poor teaching material." Medical professors prefer rapid turnover of patients to insure variability of teaching material for their students. Thus teaching hospitals, assumed to be our best hospitals, rarely admit patients for chronic treatment, or if they do, the patient is there only for a short period of time until he or she is sent to another hospital.

Chronic illness, its care, cure, and prevention, has been avoided like the plague by the medical profession. Medical management of chronic illness can be extremely time consuming. It requires little in the way of sophisticated or expensive technology. Thus the medical-industrial complex cannot profit from it and physicians cannot gain mystique and prestige from it.

Because chronic care and rehabilitative services are technologically relatively simple, what is needed more than doctors are nurses and other health workers. However, there are massive manpower shortages of health workers. At least three million additional Americans every year are left disabled, unrehabilitated, or untreated because of manpower inadequacies. *The failure to treat* these people is of course enormously costly, both financially and emotionally. Part of the failure to treat must reside in physicians' failing to transfer necessary skills to those who are capable of treating. For example, as mentioned before, there was a decade's long fight over whether doctors would allow nurses to take temperatures. If physicians continued to insist that *only* they were capable of taking temperatures, the manpower situation would be even worse. Thus the continuing and increasingly visible presence of patients with a chronic disease is threatening to the profession's monopoly control of technology. It appears as though there will never be enough physicians within the framework of our present health system. The problem of chronic disease management will be met only by a demonopolization and transfer of technology and skills to nonphysicians.

The increasing number of chronically ill people is a threat to the profession from another, but related, aspect. The medical market place for acute care is well channelized and controlled by the profession. That is, the acutely ill patient can be cared for only at a hospital, which in turn determines the size of its staff and the number of its beds. The consumer in most instances cannot choose a hospital; limitation of beds inflates their price, and only a limited number of physicians have hospital privileges. Thus supply and demand, cost and inflation, are all determined by the profession.

The situation, however, is not so simple in a nursing home or in other outpatient, chronic, or rehabilitative services where the need for technology is limited. Here it is more difficult to restrict privileges and membership and thus more difficult to channel and monopolize the patient and the medical market place.

The only role MD's have played to any serious degree in the area of chronic disease has been in their *ownership* of nursing homes, as reported by congressman David Pryor (D–Ark.) in the *Congressional Record*. This of course is an area of great profit, as well as representative of a conflict of interest. The conflict is that the more patients the physician refers to his nursing home, the more profit he makes, especially since the advent of Medicaid and Medicare. Currently there is a shortage of about one million nursing-home beds. Such shortages place beds at a premium and thus inflate their price and increase doctors' profit.

Most nursing homes, however, are nothing more than death traps—inadequately constructed and staffed, with only minimal medical supervision. Many physicians, allegedly contracted out to provide medical coverage for nursing homes, rarely showed up and when they did, performed only the most cursory of examinations. The MD's would respond more to the nurse's need for peace and quiet by abiding by the nurses' requests that patients be sedated. Many elderly patients have been overly sedated for the comfort of the nursing-home staff, only to have the sedated patients' weak respiratory muscles be incapable of responding to sedation, with the result that the patients suffocated. Oversedation is a very common cause of death in nursing homes. Even here there is some profit in oversedation; for example, noisy patients bother other patients, who complain and possibly turn business away. Noisy patients are an occupational nuisance to the staff, who are extremely hard to recruit because of the generally low salaries, other than those of physicians in the health field, and thus the physician will tend to abide by the staff's wishes.

Issues of personality and environment, individualized care and sympathy, warmth and empathy—none of these fit in with the education, training, or profits of the MD. Individualized care in many cases would involve dealing with vast social, political, and economic issues which the medical profession has studiously avoided. To confront them might expose the shortcoming of medicine, that is, that social reform and revolution have saved more lives and prevented more illness than all the doctors, drugs, and hospitals combined. Thus the profession has blatantly opposed and lobbied actively against all reforms in housing, sanitation, poverty, education, nutrition, and corporate regulation.

The only thing their training and expertise puts the modified profession in a position to know is what's best for them and not what's best for the people. Knowing which pill to prescribe for which infection doesn't qualify a physician to know what's best to charge a patient, or whether or not Congress should pass legislation to help the patient financially, or whatever. Possession of a limited amount of technology gives no one the ability, nor should it give them the right, to set overall health policy.

Nevertheless, physicians have selfishly arrogated to themselves the power of decision over all questions of health policy and medical economics. Physicians have tremendous unaccountable powers, both collectively and individaully. Collectively, they promote, practice, and police virtually the entire US health system. They exert this control at all levels, county, state, and national, through their political front or-ganization—AMPAC (American Medical Political Action Committee)—which funnels millions of dollars every year into the campaign chests of the most reactionary and racist elected officials in the country. The AMA has spent more for lobbying than any other organization in American history. In spite of representing only about 160,000 physicians, the AMA has spent far more for lobbying than has, for example, the AFL–CIO, which represents close to 16 million workers.

Through the AMA's lobbying efforts, liberal political ap-pointments to cabinet positions are successfully blocked. Thus, Dr. John Knowles never became assistant secretary of HEW (Department of Health, Education, and Welfare), and Dr. John Adriani never became the Food and Drug Admin-istration commissioner. Thus, government agencies which are supposed to protect the people and regulate the pro-fession do more to protect the profession and regulate the people. "The practice of medicine is our most critical and yet least regulated public utility," said a Dean of Harvard's Medical School. Because of such unaccountability, a license to practice medicine gives a man the right to do and to charge virtually anything, regardless of his competence. In effect the profession operates as a ruling clique with its own rules and taboos.

Just what does the word "professional" mean? It should imply that the professional person is better trained, more highly skilled, more self-disciplined, more ethical and moral, and more capable of self-policing. Unfortunately these quali-ties are just so much public relations gimmickry for making more money, for establishing doctor-dominated hierarchies, and eliminating public accountability.

Someone once described a profession as a job where you get in-service training on a lifetime, full-pay basis. Doctors attend conferences and conventions all the time. The costs involved are tax deductible as business expenses. There are enough medical conventions going on in every part of the country, almost every week, so that any vacation trip an MD might take can be a nominal attendance at a convention. Thus the vacation expenses can be written off as tax deductible and at public expense. Such are the prerogatives of a professional. The special clothes and cars are part of the image of a professional, of being privileged. The more professional one is the more unquestioning a patient will be in the physician's presence and when the bill is presented. Professionalization is nothing but a form of mysticism and serves an economic purpose for the doctor.

As pointed out elsewhere, hierarchization of the health system is both racist and male chauvinistic. That is, white, male doctors are at the top of the hierarchy while black, female aides are at the bottom. In fact, in the doctor-dominated health field it is only the MD who receives an adequate income. Virtually all other workers from nurses to aides and technicians are grossly underpaid, particularly in the face of their life and death responsibilities. Nurses and aides often have more front-line responsibilities than doctors. They certainly teach and bail out interns and residents who have had far less experience than the nurses. The health care system is really run on the backs of these underpaid people. The illness industry is the lowest paying of all industries, except for the MD who takes all the credit and profit. Robb

Burlage says the situation is like Mrs. Joan Payson's (owner of the New York Mets,) taking credit for the Mets' winning the World Series. The success of an operation or medical procedure no more belongs solely to the MD than does winning a World Series belong to Mrs. Payson or her manager. It is no coincidence that those people performing the most important social function in our society, namely, the promotion and maintenance of its health, should be among the poorest paid.

It is important to understand the framework in which the physician practices. His remuneration is directly dependent on the number and size of procedures he performs. The more he does the more he makes. But who decides what's necessary and appropriate? The profession unfortunately judges itself. The doctor's judgment is often determined by the patient's purse; for example, whether to discharge that patient, or to keep him a few days longer in the hospital, or to order a few more tests, or to do unnecessary surgery. Ultimately medical judgment is really an economic judgment.

In order to maximize profits the physician needs freedom from public scrutiny and public control and thus enthusiastically supports the "free enterprise system." However, in medicine "free enterprise" means freedom to be incompetent and freedom to charge whatever the market will bear. "Free enterprise" in medicine means each MD is a judge, jury, and all too often, executioner. In a well-functioning free enterprise system, the best are supposed to be the most rewarded. Such is not the case in our medical system. Those most rewarded are often those who can get away with the most.

In referring to the profession, Dr. Oswald Hall said: "There is a devotion to work but to work related to a specific hospital system. The development of judgment is stressed but judgment based on the advice of one's superior. The valued traits are those which can be integrated into a firmly established system of medicine. It is assumed that the person who learns to play the role will be rewarded financially and by receiving institutional prestige; it is taken for granted that there may be some delay on receiving these rewards." Thus there are purposefully numerous rungs on the hierarchial ladder in order to maintain conformity and yet encourage subservience to medical ethics and the profession. As Selig Greenberg points out: "The men with the top income and prestige are recognized as the arbiters of the system and entrusted with dispensing the rewards and administrating whatever chastisement may be called for." The laity doesn't enshrine the profession, the profession enshrines the profession. To blame mankind or the laity is to diffuse the blame and confuse the politics. The profession, as Shaw has pointed out, is indeed a "conspiracy against the laity."

Professional control of its members is often exerted through the county medical society. To get board certified one must have AMA membership and county medical society membership. Therefore without it one is denied certification and the hospital privileges which go with it. The system of control, however, is starting to break down as the university medical centers and the medical-industrial complex assume increasing power.

Failure to secure membership in a medical society means, according to the *AMA News,* an inability "to buy expensive malpractice insurance at the lower premiums that medical societies obtain by getting a master policy for their members." Professional reputations necessary for the securing of patients can be ruined by rumor and gossip by the existing members of the county medical society.

Not only does the profession have control over its own members and elect selected congressmen, but also it has successfully fought private corporations by urging boycotts of their products—for instance, the Borden Co., when its board chairman came out in favor of government support of health insurance.

Despite the professional window dressing, medical societies are basically trade union organizations whose primary function is to help their members make more money—and they have been extremely successful at it, more so than any other union.

While the medical society may use the denial of hospital admission privileges as a means of professional control and for the elimination of competition, competence is rarely a required quality to gain admission privileges. This is so, in part, because competence is extremely difficult to determine without invading the "free enterprise" of the private physician.

More important, however, is the method whereby the profession exerts economic control through the referral system. Through this system competition is regulated, interlopers are excluded, conformity is rewarded, and a rigid code of guild loyalties and professional face-saving and image-enhancing devices are enforced. As one medical educator said: "Only by adhering to the rules is an MD able to gain the recognition of his colleagues and to climb the successive rungs of the professional ladder." Since the quality of the care dispensed is often difficult to evaluate, especially by the layman, and in general ignored by the profession, there is no motivation in the system to provide quality care, and in fact a number of issues motivate against quality care, such as assembly-line office practices and profits.

The following is a letter written by a third-year medical student, Chip Smith—one year shy of his MD degree. It is a good example of how the medical student learns the specifics of the doctor-patient relationship and how that training can only tarnish that relationship.

September 2, 1969

An Open Letter to the Executive Committee of the Faculty and the Deans of the University of Pennsylvania School of Medicine.

Gentlemen:

After having successfully completed three years of your medical school's physician training program, I am leaving the school. The reason for the separation is straightforward: to continue at medical school is to continue exploiting poor people, primarily blacks, for narrow educational ends.

The doctor-patient relationship practices in your hospitals, which you expect me to honor and emulate, is a brutal relationship. It is true that everyone suffers—medical students: kept off balance, made to feel guilty about their lack of knowledge, constantly caught up in meaningless busy-work; doctors: overworked, secure only in their professional image, harassed by patients and workers whose hostility they will never understand; and patients: rich and poor alike, ignorant about their own bodies, gone haywire fearful of death, desperately struggling to believe in their white-coated saviors, trapped in an environment that is death itself made visible: sterile, efficient, uniformed, mechanical, all warmed over by the reassuring bedside-manner smile.

Everybody suffers. But the fact remains that the poor, especially blacks, suffer more.

And I've had my fill of putting it to blacks. I learned to draw blood on old black ladies. I learned to do pelvics on young black

women. I learned to do histories and physicals on black bodies
and on a few wrinkled and run down white ones. Now in order
to learn something about primary care, about long term out-pa-
tient care, I am faced again with waiting black faces in the hospital clinics. I am forced to participate in a system providing fragmented, second-rate care in the present, while loudly proclaiming
the best possible care for future patients (mostly white, suburban
folk of course . . . that is, if you don't end up having no patients
at all, as in research, public health, or administration).

Medical barbarism . . . it permeates hospital life. Needless
tests, justified on educational and experimental bases. Poorly
supervised procedures, repetitive examinations . . . "You only
learn by your mistakes," the saying goes in medical school. And
the educational principle that follows: it's OK if you make mistakes . . . the more you make, the more you learn. (And, besides,
almost all the needless pain and stress falls on charity ward patients, mostly blacks.) Endless technical discussions at the bedside,
the patient excluded except for necessary information, a piece of
meat to be thumped and prodded and exposed . . . all in the
name of high quality, scientific care. It's a farce. And a drag, and
it's brutal.

That's why I'm leaving.

II

The Doctor-Patient Relationship

INTRODUCTION

What allows the medical profession (along with the medical-industrial complex) to maintain and enhance its virtual monopoly control of the entire health system? While certain mechanisms of control are relatively clear, e.g., control of licensing, accreditation, hospital admitting privileges, and political lobbies, other means are more subtle and subjective. For example, in one sense the public at large *seems* to want to be controlled. This is particularly so in the case of the individual patient in the presence of his doctor. Here the patient is docile, dependent, and dominated. The physician is aggressive and assertive, often to the point of being hostile or cold.

The doctor-patient relationship is doctor dominated. He uses this professionally created mystique to maintain a monopolistic control of medical technology, fee determination, as well as quality and distribution of medical practice. And as mysticism allows the monopolistic control to continue, so the monopolistic control perpetuates the mysticism.

In many respects the physician cuts a uniquely potent figure. Every aspect of his demeanor contributes to this: from his business suit and businesslike manner, to his white-coated appearance of purity, cleanliness, and power, ("white coat privilege") and the omnipotence and mystery suggested by his black-magic bag.

Ironically, however, white clothing in a medical setting is quite inappropriate, especially in the operating room, where the need for good lighting produces a glare from the white uniforms. Thus, the better hospitals require that operating room clothing be green and not white.

With the black-bag suggestion that he is possessor of a vast array of technology and information, the physician purposely evokes an aura of mystery, making the patient feel that the concepts of treating illness are beyond his understanding, and that the physician need not waste his time explaining anything. Patients are encouaged to be dependent by their physicians and the health system. Augmenting the degree of oppression is the refusal of most patients to recognize and admit such dependency.

How does the above coincide with the medical ethic of "informed consent"? Informed consent means the doctor-patient relationship is to be modeled after a client-to-consultant relationship, where the people involved relate to one another as equals, not where one party acts as an uninformed, passive, inferior, unquestioning patient, and the other party as an all-knowing, authoritative mystic dealing with *your* life and death issues.

The doctor's tools, his technology, really aren't all that mysterious. They can be explained to, and understood by, the average patient. In fact, informed-consent laws demand that they be explained. But if the technology were demystified, if the patient truly understood the issues and the technology, the doctor wouldn't appear so uniquely potent and important and thus he couldn't demand spiraling inflationary fees. With unquestioning faith in the potency and efficacy of a faith healer or a physician, a patient can be influenced to pay any price asked.

Failure to inform a patient fully is literally illegal. Since virtually no patient is ever fully informed about all the drugs and procedures he ingests and endures, the basis of the doctor-patient relationship, and indeed, of most medical practices in the United States, is illegal. As technology has advanced, the doctor has increasingly used it to enhance his role of the omnipotent mystic. The more mystical he has become, the more the doctor-patient relationship diverges from the consultant-client model, which in part explains much of the increase in medical malpractice lawsuits.

TECHNOLOGY

Physicians claim to be engaged in a calling of extraordinary complexity. However, this claim is only true within a limited context. After all, a general physician can learn in six to twelve months the technology to diagnose and treat 90 per cent of the disease situations he encounters. The overwhelming health problem in the United States is the long-term treatment of chronic diseases, such as, high blood pressure, diabetes, heart disease, neurosis, obesity, and senility. Such treatment, however, requires so little technology that a few university medical centers have trained successfully nurse-clinicians to treat and manage these patients with a fraction of the training doctors receive and at a fraction of the expense. That is, the nurse is trained to perform some aspects of the physical examination, such as a medical history, to interpret laboratory studies and prescribe a treatment, though nominally, at least, under the supervision of an MD. What is complex, however, is the implementation of programs, providing comprehensive health care to all who need it—and we all do eventually.

"Implementation" means where, when, how, and with what to obtain, coordinate, and integrate nursing homes, hospitals, clinics. That's a relatively complex problem of administration. The medical problem of examination, diagnosis, and treatment of chronically ill patients, however, is relatively simple. But in admitting this simplicity, the medical profession would remove a rationalization for the maintenance of their high fees.

Only the medical profession opposed the broad scale implementation of programs such as the nurse-clinician program, in spite of their being of equal quality to traditional programs, and much cheaper. This sort of opposition makes the implementation complex. It is this kind of a politico-economic complexity that is often difficult to understand, and not the complexity of the doctors' tools and technology. For example, medical care is a commodity offered for sale to those who can afford it, and yet it is also a service dedicated (at least in theory) to be rendered to all those who need it. It is the incongruities of the delivery of medical service which are most complex.

While there have been numerous technological advances, very few of them have any relevance to, or correlation with, the improvements in our morbidity or mortality rates. For example, open-heart surgery, no matter how glamorous a procedure it might be, has saved very few lives. Doctors would like us to believe that they are responsible for the major advances in health in the last couple of centuries, when, in fact, the major advances have been produced by social reforms and revolutions. The improvements in nutrition, sanitation, housing, and so on, have allowed far more people to live longer and healthier than any single discovery in medical technology or combination of them. Actually, in the last ten years, the period of the greatest number of major advances in scientific medical discoveries, the life expectancy rate in the United States has remained virtually unchanged, while in twenty other countries the rate has lengthened. Again the "progress" has been used to increase the doctor's armament of mysticism rather than implement and provide for health care to the general public.

George Bernard Shaw described his image of medical "progress" as "Science at the Prow and Commerce at the Helm" and then accused doctors for being "unscientific" about their science when it interfered with their commerce.

For the medical student, whose education is filled with much misplaced emphasis on a wide range of sciences, including biochemistry, physiology, biophysics, genetics, pharmacology, microbiology, and electronics, it is difficult to see people as people but only as biochemical machines. Such emphasis on the hard sciences is totally disproportionate, especially if it means neglecting the humanities and social sciences. However, it is economically advantageous to the doctor to emphasize technology, organic diseases, pathology, and the like over the social sciences and public health. From such emphasis on "technology and science" evolves a very basic sense of the impersonality of medical care. Doctors are too busy simply to talk to people.

The demand and need for the doctor's medical services far exceed the supply, allowing the physician to choose his patients and their treatments. Along the lines of maximum financial benefit, he spends as little time as possible with cases complicated by emotional, social, or economic factors and avoids home visits, especially night visits, which are all too time consuming. And "time is money." Spending time consoling a patient who recently had a death in the family and is now suffering from depression and anxiety which exacerbate an ulcer and produces headaches prevents the physician from seeing a greater number of patients. It's much quicker and more economical to prescribe aspirin and warm milk than to get at the roots of the depression by giving emotional warmth and support to the patient.

This failure to deal with patients as people with human emotions, rather than as physiological machines continues despite the fact that numerous studies have shown that a minimum of 75 per cent of patients in a doctor's office have emotional problems complicating their physiological problems, and at least 25 per cent of the patients have nothing but emotional problems.

Doctors are extremely quick to recommend and rely on expensive laboratory tests and procedures. Again "science and technology" prevail. The laboratory test is often seen as more precise diagnostically and thus more "scientific." However, such rationalizations become more insignificant when compared with the economic determinants of overreliance on the use of the laboratory.

With the need to see and examine as many patients as quickly as possible, the MD does the shortest possible physical examination and history taking. Because the history and physical are so cursory, the MD is increasingly dependent upon laboratory tests to back him up in case he's missed anything. A reliance on lab tests has other advantages. Physicians often own or have stock in the laboratory which does their testing. Thus, the physician has an investment in over-testing his patients. Some physicians often have a kickback arrangement with the laboratory, where the referring physician is paid 10 or 20 per cent of the lab bill. Other physicians simply pay the lab bill themselves and then prepare a separate, more expensive, lab bill for the patient.

The technology of the laboratory adds to the mystique of the physician. The doctor appears to be the possessor of a vast array of knowledge and power—and in a sense, he is. After all, only physicians can order medical laboratory tests. Thus, physicians define themselves by the degree to which they have monopoly control of a medical setting and situation and by the degree to which they can gain profit and privilege from that monopoly control. Lab tests have the aura of objective scientific finality, when, in fact, many lab tests are often quite inaccurate, unnecessarily expensive to the patient, and require a great deal of subjective interpretation. They also have a wide range of false positive and false negative values.

The most efficient and profitable form of industrial or medical practice appears to be the assembly line. It is in this setting where a maximum degree of technology can be applied in the shortest period of time, truly creating an illness industry.

Even assembly-line practices can add to a physician's mystique. The patient must assume that if the doctor can do a history and physical, diagnose and prescribe a treatment, all in a ten- to fifteen-minute period, the doctor, indeed, must be an incredibly, even magically, skilled professional.

Assembly-line practices and cursory examinations leave the physician in a state of considerable ignorance about the patient. To overcome this ignorance the doctor will not only overrely on lab tests, but will also overrely on referring the patient to another physician, to uncover what he was too busy to notice, diagnose, or treat. Referrals also produce kickbacks for and referrals back to the original physician. One physician's assembly-line practice generates referrals to another physician's assembly-line practice. By multiple referrals the original referring doctor is, as are all subsequent doctors, legally covered. Each original diagnosis, treatment, and so on, is "confirmed" by each new physician.

Unfortunately, multiple referrals not only greatly inflate the cost of medical care, they highly fragment the care as well. Ultimately, no single physician assumes primary responsibility for the care of the patient. Each physician in the referring network assumes that a physician other than himself is assuming primary responsibility. Thus, the accountability and liability of each individual physician is lessened considerably. How can a physician be sued for neglect or malpractice if the patient has been referred to three or four physicians, with each physician claiming that the previous MD or the next MD is the one to blame? The rapid rise in negligence and malpractice suits brought to court is in part a reflection of the increase in numbers of referring doctors people are seeing. Concomitant with this increase is fragmentation, irresponsibility, unaccountability, and thus liability.

To spend more time with a patient and less time with medical technology may deemphasize the technology and its accompanying mysticism. When people are sick and feel helpless and afraid, they tend to regress into childlike dependency. Under such circumstances they often welcome a doctor's authoritarian qualities which they might otherwise resent. This dependency is encouraged by the doctor, as such a patient is more unquestioning, "things run smoother," the doctor can manipulate the treatment program as he wishes, that is, order more lab tests, make more referrals, shorten or prolong the time spent in expensive hospital beds, prescribe more drugs, charge higher fees, and answer fewer of the questions the patient might ask.

In spite of the rapid rise in medical malpractice suits, nowhere near the real number of potential suits has been brought to court. Numerous negligent physicians have avoided the courtroom either because of a warm, trusting, doctor-patient relationship or a successful use of their technological monopoly and mysticism to encourage patient dependency and apparent satisfaction, or fear. Such physicians create in patients a need to believe that their physician has indeed performed a miracle. How else could he justify the financial burden he then places on his patient?

One of the inherent contradictions in rising technology and its concomitant rising mysticism is a consequential increase of patient expectation for rising levels in quality, quantity, diversity, and accessibility of health care. However, there is an increasing disparity between what seems to be promised by the technology, e.g., heart- and lung-transplant procedures, and what is actually delivered, e.g., an inability to deal with and provide for senility, alcoholism, addiction, common colds, ambulance and outpatient services. We have the technology to get an astronaut to the moon, but we can't get an ambulance to take the patient to the hospital. Mass media plays up medical advances, adding both to the MD's mystique and appearance of omniscience. However, in reality the MD can't or won't meet these expectations. This can raise the patient's sense of alienation and increase his opposition to the health system.

What little research is done is more for institutional and professional prestige, profit, and prerogative than for implementable, therapeutic discoveries. That research which appears most spectacular is supported and enhanced by mass media coverage. Surgical heart transplantation and the like get international media coverage. The inevitable funerals which follow, do not. It's not as entertaining as the operation, and the function of news is much more to entertain than it is to inform. Thus the public expects more and gets relatively less.

Medical technology in general and the drug industry in particular place a great deal of emphasis on the concept of "a magic pill for every ill." Such reliance on drugs not only supports the pharmaceutical industry, but allows the physician to appear objective, scientific, and exact.

It's the authority to dispense the magic pill which gives an MD his rationalized authority and superiority over, say, a Ph.D. By enhancing the aura of potency around pills, a physician enhances his mystique as the only one fully trained to prescribe and evaluate medication and thus to control all medical care, when in reality the dispensing of pills is only a relatively minor part of health care.

Many physicians have an educated distaste for admitting that they don't know something. Primarily, however, it's an economic distaste—to not know is to lose the image of omniscience. Here, too, drugs fit in. To prescribe a pill—any pill—has the appearance of omniscience. After all, who can imagine a doctor prescribing the wrong pill—even if it's a placebo? Yet, in fact, many drugs are prescribed more to treat the physician's image than the patient's illness.

Even prescription writing is a form of mysticism. Not only is the mysticism in the form of a secret message between doctor and druggist, but the message is often illegible and partly in Latin. Contrary to "informed consent" ethics and legislation, many physicians admit not wanting their patients to know what has been prescribed for them.

The prescription necessary for the purchase of many drugs would not be needed if health care were readily accessible. If a health system is responsive to people's needs, people won't look outside of that system to meet their needs. They wouldn't attempt to treat themselves by going to a drugstore and purchasing over-the-counter medicine (as opposed to prescription medicine) and they wouldn't go to chiropractors or quacks. Prescriptions are another way of preserving a dual system of health care.

If a doctor-patient relationship is a warm, supportive, equal, and constructive one, doctor and patient will arrive at a mutually satisfactory treatment plan, for which no prescription would ever be necessary. It's only when the physician or health service is inaccessible and the doctor-patient relationship is no longer a mutual one, that prescriptions become necessary. The use of prescriptions in modern medical practice is a measure of the degree to which that practice is fragmented, alienating, or nonexistent.

Prescriptions are functionally a form of channelization and social control of the patient. That is, in order to get the medicine, the patient must go to the doctor to get the prescription and then to the druggist. Under *current circumstances* I wouldn't be in favor of abolishing the prescription system. However, the prescription system does emphasize that when accessibility is limited, when doctors spend very little time per patient in an assembly-line practice, they become increasingly reliant on mechanical devices such as prescriptions to control the patient market place. When health care is maximally accessible, when the health system itself is not so alien, then illness behavior assumes an entirely different picture. Compliance with a treatment plan increases where care is accessible and comprehensive, where the doctor-patient relationship is a humane one and not a mechanical one.

Another contradiction is emerging. As the general society becomes increasingly dependent on technology, people become more socially alienated, needing further emotional and supportive modalities from the health system. The system in turn is giving less and less because of the increasing manpower shortages and a greater emphasis on the more profitable assembly-line care. More and more dissatisfaction provides increased demands for consumer control. Yet meeting individual needs would expose the inadequacies of the present medical system, showing it to be an illness-removal system, rather than a health-enhancement system, where physicians would have less prestige and profits.

Assembly-line practices also lead to millions of unnecessary surgical operations, some of which are fatal. If a woman comes in complaining of irregular periods, it's much simpler and more profitable to do a hysterectomy, ("exorcism by surgery") than to take a long history and do a careful examination.

Any new system of health care must deal with the manpower issue to avoid physicians' working a sixty-hour week in an assembly-line practice. Manpower needs must be calculated closer to a thirty-five-hour week and to a more individualized medical practice. The profession may claim the United States has "the best medical care in the world"—but the question remains, for whom, how many, and how often?

Far less than half the population has what could be called a personal or family physician, someone who is completely familiar with the person and his family not only in medical terms but in possessing a total awareness of their life style and needs. Having a family or personal physician means having a physician whom one sees regularly and not simply at times of acute emergencies. Anything short of this could not be called a personal or family physician. A minimum of one-third of Americans, when they see a physician at all, see him only in impersonal clinics or hospital wards and not in private offices or homes. One hundred and thirty counties in the United States have no physicians whatsoever. Such is the degree of our manpower problem.

To burden the physician with a need to develop an intimate relationship with his patient is to burden him with what he considers an economic hardship. Before the advent of modern technology, the doctor-patient relationship and the doctor's treatment were primarily words. The advent of technology eliminated the economic need for most of those words. There were new areas and methods by which a patient could be charged. Thus, in changing from his practice of words to technology, the doctor went from a witch doctor economic relationship to an urban technological one, with a consequent rise in income.

It's more profitable for the doctor to deal with the abnormality and technology of a specific organ than to deal with the overall functioning of an individual. In a sense doctors are more interested in the trouble than in those who are in trouble. And the treatment of the trouble pays off. It can be done cheaply and quickly.

No one talks to the patient; no one loses any time. Or money. Such physicians will tell a patient: "There's nothing wrong with you; it's just your nerves." In this manner the physician avoids many fee-losing hours and unprofitable conversation. As a token of support and interest the doctor may offer a tranquilizer. Many physicians rationalize their curtness by seeing all emotionally related symptoms as malingering, and malingering is antithetical to a work-oriented, work-valued, success-oriented, profit-driven society.

The more sophisticated and clever physician learns how to give the impression that he could give the patient an hour and then pacifies him with a few minutes. Such is not the keystone of an honest, open, informed relationship. To attempt to satisfy people under these terms is to use medicine as a tool of oppression.

Under such circumstances it's difficult to believe the sincerity of the medical profession when they speak of the "sacredness of the doctor-patient relationship." A relationship characterized by assembly-line practices and multiple referrals can hardly be characterized as "sacred" when a patient spends more time with a tube of blood, than a talk with his physician. What is sacred from the doctor's point of view is his freedom to manipulate that relationship to his own lucrative advantage. In order to preserve his control and freedom to manipulate, he and his profession do everything possible to keep out "outsiders," such as government and community review boards.

An important implication of the "sacredness" of the doctor-patient relationship is "confidentiality." The communication between doctor and patient is "privileged." Yet, in 1969, when university medical centers such as Yale-New Haven Hospital computerized all their medical records on a centralized city computer, readily accessible to police and other investigatory agencies, the medical profession never questioned this invasion of privacy and confidentiality. In fact it is the medical-industrial complex which supports computerization and centralization of all the records and data of all service agencies, e.g., police, education, welfare, and so forth. The computer manufacturers of the medical-industrial complex are attempting to use health as a market arena and are unconcerned about confidentiality. All too often doctors and hospitals freely hand patients' medical records over to police officials upon their verbal request, even though a bullet wound, et al., is the only legitimate reason for involving the police.

On the other hand, the ethic of confidentiality is often used to the physician's advantage. For example, a patient who wishes to sue his physician suddenly finds his medical records so confidential that he, himself, cannot see them. This is hardly a paradigm of an informed, open, "sacred" relationship.

There simply are no reasons why patients should not be allowed to see their own charts and records. There are no ethical, medical, or legal reasons—only economic reasons—to protect the secrecy and sanctity of the doctor's technology, to avoid exposing an error he may have committed, thus opening himself up to lawsuits, and to insure that a maximum degree of mystery and mystique enshrouds the doctor-patient relationship.

However, there are many reasons for allowing, and indeed, encouraging patients to *see and understand* their medical records. It allows the patient to be fully informed and thus to realistically consent to all procedures and prescriptions relevant to him. The patient can also correct any misconceptions or errors the physician might have made concerning the patient's medical history or symptoms.

Interference in the "sacred" doctor-patient relationship has been used as a scare tactic by the profession to oppose any progressive legislation which might help the patient, but in some way interfere with the physician's monopoly control. The profession has articulated its opposition to "interference" in the doctor-patient relationship as no "third-party" schemes. Thus, the profession has opposed Blue Cross, group practice, Medicare, Social Security, public immunization, venereal disease clinics, school health services, and Red Cross blood banks. Thus, the profession has opposed anything which might impinge on their total unaccountability in any way—all in the name of protecting the doctor-patient relationship.

Physicians in 1964 were so fearful of third-party intervention from the impending passage of the Medicare program that they threatened a national strike. That is, they were blackmailing the public by threatening to withhold lifesaving services. In 1962 they spent over $5 million, according to the *Washington Post,* just to defeat this particular piece of legislation. The profession has gone to the extreme of promoting the belief that "third parties" are voyeurs who will come into the doctor's office to watch him examine a patient to see that he does it correctly.

Promoting "sacredness" of the doctor-patient relationship, as an attempt to keep out "third parties," is also a rationalization to insure maintenance of the fee-for-service system. Likewise, the profession opposes physicians on fixed salaries, just as in prepaid group and hospital practices. Physicians on fixed salaries are not dependent on a medical market place controlled by the county medical society, and thus are not readily controlled by the AMA's county medical society.

They are also less likely to pay their AMA membership dues, let alone join the AMA. Proposed government health-insurance schemes have attempted to place physicians on salaries and thus have been opposed by the AMA. Because group and hospital practices have their own sources of referrals and patient pools, these physicians are also independent of the county medical society's referral network.

Fixed salaries do not maximize income for the individual physician and thus have been opposed on this ground as well. New services under the present system are added and promoted in the most profitable fee-for-service fashion, rather than in the most economical and serviceable way. Thus the tacked-on nature of services gives the medical system its appearance of anarchy.

Fee-for-service is part of the free-enterprise ethic. The physician charges one fee to a patient without insurance. If the patient should get insurance, he'll be charged a higher fee, so that he pays the same amount, but in addition to what the insurance company already pays the physician. All of this maximizes profit and inflates the price of health, as well as the price of insurance.

The profession has complained that any alteration in the fee-for-service system of payments is unethical, because it would ruinously alter the doctor-patient relationship.

There has been considerably less concern shown for this relationship when the patient has no fees because he or she is too poor to pay—in fact, the patient foregoes the entire relationship. All too often the patient is relegated to the charity hospital and its clinics to be treated by an MD or a student he never saw before and probably never will again. And if all those who need health care ever got to a clinic, they would overwhelm it, making it difficult to see any physician even once, thus making an absurdity of the doctor-patient relationship.

The AMA even opposed legislation which would have allowed free inoculations with the Salk vaccine, in spite of the fact that unless it was free, millions of children would be denied access to it or delayed in receiving it. The AMA's rationalization for opposition was that health care should go through "regular channels," i.e., "ethical channels," and not dispensed without a fee-for-service.

While the conservatives of the medical profession, the individualistic entrepreneurs fight for the retention of fees-for-services, the liberals of the medical-industrial complex, "the corporatists," prefer fixed salaries, which would make the system more predictable and thus better fit for corporate management. But the struggle is not simply over professional ethics, but rather over who will have access to the patient's pocketbook.

The introduction of Medicaid and other payment innovations will simply increase the demand for services without increasing the supply and redistribution of physicians and facilities. Short-supply and heavy-demand economics will produce an inflationary spiral, placing increased strain on physicians and facilities. No publicly accountable price or service controls will encourage doctors to spend even less time with patients and to charge even more. The tendency to charge more and more will be exacerbated if Medicaid and the like will pay whatever is "reasonable cost," since whatever is "reasonable" will be determined by the local medical society. Clearly, to break this cycle, a greater amount of manpower and facilities are needed, utilizing nonphysician review boards. Quality control, policy setting, licensing, and accreditation all must belong to the consumer and not to the profession or the corporate medical-industrial complex. Simply "advancing" medical science and technology alone hardly changes anything for the better.

The more technological medicine becomes, the greater will be the patient's bewilderment and dependency over what is actually happening to him. Thus it is to the profession's advantage to increase at least the appearance of complexity in medicine. This is partly done by the unnecessary use of highly centralized, imposing glass and steel medical centers. The imposing aura of greatness and magnitude is enough to scare the unsophisticated patient into submission. In fact, numerous studies have shown that the size and structure of the hospital literally does scare people away, until it is too late, and their diseases have advanced beyond repair. Decentralized, small facilities would be less formidable, more visible, accessible, and welcoming. They would eliminate some of the imposing mystical aura of hospitals, their unwieldy bureaucracy, and thus some of their inaccessibility, unaccountability, and buck passing. People talk about an inability to "fight City Hall," but that is nothing in comparison to getting satisfaction from a monolithic hospital. The situation is considerably different at a local, decentralized, and personalized clinic where all but the very complicated, and thus rarely used, facilities and equipment are located.

Patients are not only intimidated by awe-inspiring medical centers, but also by the disparity in income and status between themselves and their physicians. The patient is thus less critical and less expectant of the common decency and civility from his doctor that would allow an equal and mutual relationship to develop. Intimidated patients are occasionally literally afraid to go to the doctor's office. A real class and often racial antagonism develops. The physician moves to the suburbs, not only to increase his access to a wealthier clientele, but also to comfort himself by minimizing the class and racial antagonisms of his practice. Thus large segments of both rural and urban populations have no access to a family or personal physician.

As a physician's clientele become wealthier, the more arrogant he becomes toward his less financially fortunate patients. He no longer needs them in any context.

The depersonalization and alienation of the doctor-patient relationship, the physician shortage, and the physician's shortage of time have led more patients to seek help from nonphysician sources such as quacks, spiritualists, and chiropractors. While the quacks may be short on technology, they do offer the patient at least a personal relationship. The medical profession doesn't oppose chiropractors just on the basis of their lack of technical efficacy, but on the basis of their competition for a room in the medical market place. And given the fact that 20 per cent of most GP patients are suffering from purely emotional upsets, the quack probably does a better job treating them than does the average MD. All of which says that quacks are as successful as they are because they fill needs not met by the health system. When those needs are met, there will be no room and no need for quacks.

It isn't the development of technology per se that has interfered with a quality doctor-patient relationship, but rather, the fact that physicians no longer need that relationship to maximize their profits. Too much blame is placed on technology, rather than on those who use and control it.

Technology is abused by the profession to create more impersonal, assembly-line practices, while technology itself is neutral. The controllers of medical policy, the profession and the medical-industrial complex, determine the setting for, and application of, the technology. Simply decreasing the amount of technology, in and of itself, won't change anything; only medical policy control under consumer regulation will. The science and art of medicine are not intrinsically incompatible. What is incompatible is the use of illness and its treatment as a profit-making marketable commodity, where that market is promoted, policed, and protected by an unaccountable profession and the corporate interests of the medical-industrial complex. This basic conflict will only be resolved by consumer control.

While the frequent failure of communication between physician and patient is one of the great dilemmas in medicine, quality comprehensive health care remains a greater one. The profession doesn't have an image problem just because of bad communication techniques. It's ridiculous to talk about the image problem of the doctor, or the communication problem of the doctor and patient, or the sacredness of the doctor-patient relationship, when millions literally have no doctor. The profession is more concerned with its image than its substance.

The AMA has spent over the last decade *tens of millions of dollars* on public relations to promote the professional appearance of unselfish service to humanity and adherence to professional ideals. The more idealistic the physician appears, the less likely is the confident patient to question his fees. It isn't just the doctor's ego which is fed when he looks like the knight in shiny white coat; it's his pocketbook.

For the physician, there simply is no profit in looking after his patient's welfare—provided he isn't caught not looking. Malpractice suits, particularly successful ones, have done more to raise standards of medical practice than have major technical advances in medical care. For example, malpractice suits have forced many physicians to:

1. Understand and become aware of the contraindications of certain drugs.

2. Be fully versed on all the material in a patient's medical chart.

3. Keep clear, intelligible medical records in order to have a much better and accessible picture of the patient's medical history and treatment (and better support in the event of a lawsuit).

4. Be aware of a patient's allergic history. This has saved thousands of lives from death by allergic reactions to penicillin.

Actually, the above examples appear to be totally common-sensical. What could be more reasonable than to expect an MD to understand the side effects of a drug or to take complete histories of his patients? Yet thousands of doctors, tens of thousands of times, didn't, until the people sued for malpractice and began making at least part of the system accountable.

The economic evolution of health care removes the physician further and further away from the patient's life. What had formerly been a private relationship between two individuals has been reshaped into a major industry, involving some fifty medical specialties and subspecialties and more than seventy ancillary technical occupations. As a result, the physician knows less and less about the patient's life. Yet, conditions in the home, job, and community are often extremely important determinants of someone's illness. For instance, is a man's heart condition aggravated by having to climb stairs, working long hours, being harrangued by the boss, and strained by long rides to work? The MD must be able to account for all these factors, while he is less and less likely and able to do so. Seeing a patient in a hospital bed is infinitely different from seeing him in the context of his home, family, and community. Emotional, social, and economic issues are increasingly involved in the cause and cures of medical problems, but the physician is, in many ways, hiding from these issues behind his desk and his white coat.

FEES

Assembly-line medical services are, of course, financially meaningless to the physician without a fee for each service. As the most protected aspect of the United States medical system, the sacredness of the doctor-patient relationship is really a code term for the sacredness of the fee-for-service system.

A patient will come to the physician's office complaining of a cough. The doctor may or may not listen to the patient's history and chest. He will hand him a prescription for cough medicine or an antibiotic and send him home or to work. The service is a brief one and the patient has a 90 per cent chance of getting better. The odds are good for the patient, in spite of the doctor's superficial interest. The quality of care, however, is poor, because no one knows the diagnosis. The careful and concerned physician will take a thorough and time-consuming history, undress the patient, use the stethescope, order necessary tests to arrive at a diagnosis, and then and only then prescribe an appropriate therapy.

Fee splitting is essentially "buying and selling the sick with their own money." It not only inflates the costs, but also promotes needless surgery. The fee splitting and kickback referral processes are particularly accentuated in the relation-

ship between general practitioners and surgeons. The disparity in income between surgeon and GP is greatest between
these two types of practices. As has been noted, the GP's are
bitter about this disparity; they are excluded from the hospital
and from doing the surgery they are potentially capable of
doing. Their bitterness leads them to demand kickbacks. On
the other hand, there are surgeons who can only maintain a
practice through a referral system and network. It is rare for
a patient to go directly to a surgeon without a referral. Thus,
surgeons are dependent on, and have no choice (even though
most are more than willing) but to participate in, a kickback
system, especially if they have just opened an office.

GP's are often fearful of making a referral. They may lose
the patient. Thus many GP's, finding it necessary to make a
referral, will send the patient to a specialist in a city as far
removed from him as possible, rather than to a local specialist, who might "keep" or "steal" the patient.

An even more dramatic kickback arrangement is seen in
the variant of the case of general practitioners who are fearful of losing patients to surgeons. The GP may try to control the patient market place by doing the surgery himself—
often incompetently, because of lack of continuous surgical
experience. An even more perverse aspect is "ghost surgery."
Here the GP examines, diagnoses, and recommends surgery
to the patient. The GP then appears in the operating room
prepared to do the surgery. However, while the patient is
under anesthesia, a real surgeon enters the room and performs the actual operation. By "ghosting," the GP retains his
control of the clientele. Aside from the inflationary nature
of this procedure, two physicians instead of one, it's medically
risky. The surgeon performing the operation will not be able

to do a proper preoperative evaluation on the patient, nor a postoperative follow-up—both of which are necessary to insure adequate continuity of care.

Those surgeons and GP's who aren't engaged in fee splitting, kickbacks, and other unethical activities aid and abet these practices by their conspiracy of silence, often enforced by the county medical society.

Pathologists frequently cooperate with those doing unnecessary surgery. By approving lab reports which state that the removed tissue is diseased, when, in fact, it isn't, pathologists abet unnecessary surgery. For such cooperative pathologists an additional fee is given.

Once a normal organ is removed, the stage is set for a second surgical procedure. The first procedure often results in tissue adhesions which, at a later date will produce abdominal pain, giving the surgeon, or GP, or whoever the operator happens to be, an excuse for additional surgery and additional profit.

Again, the moral is the more services performed, the more fees collected. Numerous, though often unnecessary hysterectomies have been called the "rape of the pelvis." Close to 40 per cent of all hysterectomies done in the last ten years are unjustifiable on medical or surgical grounds. Another procedure called "uterine suspension" is often done under the rationalization that it helps relieve backache. Fully 90 per cent of such operations are unnecessary, and worse, produce no symptomatic relief, except for the medical profession. Dr. Martin Cherkasky's study of the Teamsters Union reveals that a minimum of 20 per cent of their hospital admissions were totally unnecessary. It is not enough to blame a few evil or greedy physicians for these misdeeds; this practice is rampant throughout the profession. The medical system promotes and encourages such corruption, as does our profit-oriented economy.

"Tissue committees" which are strong and responsive to patient needs have produced dramatic drops in surgical procedures, often cutting some operative procedures to one-third of previous levels. Unfortunately there is little incentive for the hospital or its staff to develop such committees and when they do, they are often composed of the doctors doing most of the unnecessary surgery.

Such abuses as unnecessary surgery are not confined to a few hospitals but rather, as a past president of the American College of Surgeons has said, ". . . exist in the majority of hospitals in the United States today." Besides, it's fiscally important to the hospital to keep its beds filled nearly to capacity. Unnecessary surgery makes no difference in the hospital's financial records, except to improve them. Under the current system there is no way to insure that a tissue committee will be more responsive to patient needs than to professional needs. It's more likely to be the latter than the former, as that is where the profits lie.

Kickback arrangements can be developed in a variety of settings, not necessarily limited to other physicians. A profitable conspiracy can be worked out with druggists, opticians, technicians, laboratories, and ambulance companies. Connections with these enterprises encourage their overutilization in order to reap additional profits and tend to inflate the price of health. For example, a number of years ago opticians' kickbacks to physicians forced up the retail price of eyeglasses by at least 25 per cent. The price inflation of glasses reached such scandalous proportion in some areas that the United

States Department of Justice had to step in to end the most flagrant and profitable aspects of this practice.

Numerous New York State investigating agencies have repeatedly exposed a considerable degree of collusion between doctors and ambulance-chasing lawyers. The doctor-lawyer teams bilk insurance companies by heavy padding or completely fraudulent bills in accident cases. In the New York City area alone it was noted that thirteen hundred physicians were involved. One official from the Attorney General's Office described the extent of the racket as "staggering the imagination." Numerous other New York State and City investigations revealed widespread fees for mythical services, kickbacks, and the like.

Hospitals do have a minor problem maintaining their unaccountability compared with office medical practice; what goes on in the hospital is more readily observable and potentially accountable than what goes on in the private office. Since most procedures involve nurses, aides, technicians, assistants, and other physicians, there aren't many secrets within the hospital, although the nuances never reach the public.

The surgeons may bury their mistakes, but others refer theirs to some cooperative specialists or business. An even more ominous conflict of interest is seen in the case of the undertakers or morticians who control the ambulance services in many cities. What could motivate them to provide quick, medically appropriate ambulance services, if they own the local mortuary and stand to gain far more from the patient's death than his health?

Iatrogenic diseases and disabilities (those caused by the doctor) are one of the commonest causes of poor health and death. Much of the pathology induced by the doctor is derived from the medical-economic settings and policies which encourage it. Such settings and policies encourage assembly-line practices, overmedication, overreferral, fragmented care, unnecessary surgery, failure to do adequate histories and physicals, and thus overdependence on lab procedures, none of which are without some risk. The greater the advances of technology, whether it be drugs or surgical procedures, the greater the risk of iatrogenic disease and death. For example, virtually every drug has its side effects. Virtually all have killed people at one time or another.

Not surprisingly, by 1949 the United States National Office of Vital Statistics instituted the listing of a new cause-of-death category, namely: "Deaths ascribed to therapeutic misadventure as primary causes." Of course the number of deaths attributable to such causes is always grossly understated, as few physicians would be willing to report deaths based on their own mistakes. Within the present system physicians can create disease as easily as they can cure it, and often do, given the profit motivation of the system. A medical professor puts it that medical education fails to emphasize that ". . . knowing when not to treat is fully as important as knowing when to treat." But the system is geared for overtreatment, overutilization of services, and overreferral, all of which result in the misuse and abuse of technology. So the doctor who wishes to spend as little time as possible with the patient is obliged to give him something for his money, even if it is just a prescription, a procedure, a test, or a referral—to placate him and profit from him.

Since careful histories are tedious and time consuming, it's more expedient for the doctor to experiment with medication to see which one, if any, will ultimately work. Thus the patient is forced to return for additional brief and profitable visits.

Physicians are trained to concentrate on disease and pathology. But aside from creating an atmosphere where prevention and enhancement are neglected, the concentration on pathology also creates negative suggestions to the patient's mind. For example: Around 70 per cent of patients who visit a cardiologist are suffering from exaggerated, unnecessary anxiety about their hearts, arising from careless or unconsidered remarks of doctors. A poor doctor-patient relationship, the physician's need for an assembly-line practice and his emphasis on profits from disease and not health are largely responsible for such a condition. Thus, anxiety about one's heart and any concomitant disability is often iatrogenically created.

Since the physician alone has the privilege, power, and authority to define illness and since he alone can determine (legally) when the patient is well, the line between the necessary and the unnecessary visit, procedure, appliance, lab test, referral, and operation is extremely difficult to draw. That's the point of mystification, control of technology and education. If only the doctor knows, only he can control the market. Thus, as one medical writer observed: "Some doctors have a distaste for terminating a source of income and thus keep patients coming back for procedures that either are worthless or could just as well be taken care of at home."

The quality of care a patient receives is, to a large degree, determined by his ability to pay the physician. The physician will spend less time with the poor patient, give him a less thorough history and physical examination, and avoid ordering necessary tests, procedures, and referrals. With the advent of Medicaid and Medicare the situation is often changed.

The patient is now somewhat subsidized. The MD will see the patient the same number of minutes, but perhaps more often, ordering unnecessary tests, procedures, and referrals. As long as it's paid for, whether by the patient or the government, the physician can profit from it.

If the patient has only standard hospital insurance, that is, little or no coverage for outpatient or office procedures, a great incentive exists to hospitalize the patient. This means that the doctor will often delay care until the patient is sick enough to merit admission to a hospital, where his bills can then be paid. As a result, relatively minor symptoms are allowed to progress into major ones, occasionally with fatal results.

The other side of overdoing procedures, treatment, and prescribing is failing to do enough of the appropriate action, e.g., adequate history and physical, and adequate preoperative workup. Numerous brain tumors are missed because of failure to do what should be routine, i.e., a neurological examination. The delay in diagnosis is often fatal to the patient, but costs the doctor nothing.

It's simpler and more profitable for the doctor to prescribe the wrong treatment, forcing the patient to return, than to take the time to make the right diagnosis. There's no profit in curing, only in treating—and treating—and treating. This situation has been documented time and time again in professional journals, which are not readily accessible to the public. Studies in New Orleans, North Carolina, and Washington document cases where delays in diagnosis and thus delays in the appropriate treatment proved fatal, while the original doctor *treated* and *treated*—incorrectly—when a little more time to elicit all the symptoms and signs, and to do the appropriate tests, would have saved patients' lives. In a New

Orleans study only 15 per cent of the patients were treated promptly and appropriately. In a North Carolina study only 17 per cent had received an adequate physical examination. In a Washington study 70 per cent of the patients were delayed in finding the right treatment and care. The above cases are not exceptions, but the rule. As a result of the above, there is greater disparity between what physicians are positively and constructively capable of performing and what they actually do. Thus, malpractice suits have risen dramatically. One in every six physicians has been sued at least once for malpractice.

There is a correlation between frequency of malpractice suits and areas where the highest surgical fees are charged. In one sense lawsuits are derived from the failure of physicians to meet expected needs. Surgery has the most channelized and controlled market. There is far more mystique, excitement, and ultimate expense surrounding the surgeon than any other specialist. Thus, when results don't meet expectations, the likelihood of a lawsuit is greater.

If every patient who has suffered malpractice sued his physician, there would probably be at least three times the number of suits now present. The lack of more suits is in part due to the way in which patients are intimidated, pacified, and mystified by the doctor. This is in great part maintained by a lack of any third party, particularly consumer, intervention, and supervision.

The profession likes to create and maintain the myth that the overall general problems of health care are beyond the comprehension of laymen. The term "layman" is used as a synonym for "moron." The editor of the medical journal *Modern Hospital* said: "A doctor who objects to lay interference . . . is asking the medical profession to be given the status of an untouchable priesthood. . . ." The priesthood concept, whether it applies to the church or to the medical profession, is against the concept of accountability, democracy, and an informed constituency.

A number of public opinion surveys in recent years have shown that most people find little fault with their doctors, but ironically, have a less favorable opinion of the medical profession as a whole and doctors in general. To me, as a psychiatrist, it sounds as though the American patient population have repressed their anger at their particular physicians —an anger created by the dependent position he has placed them in, and which he maintains them in for economic benefit. The repressed patient isn't aware of his oppression. The effects of mysticism diffuse the anger against the physician and direct it toward the great unknown of the "medical profession" or the "medical system."

While, in a very real sense, blame and anger should be directed against the medical system, the thought of an individual patient taking on a system is, to say the least, intimidating. It's structured to be that way. Historically and culturally we've been trained to respond individually and not collectively, and of course isolated individual assaults on a system as powerful and prestigious as the medical system have provided no meaningful way in which it can be held accountable, to be dealt with quickly and justly. Unquestionably, fees keep patients away from doctors and hospitals. They are a roadblock to health and make a mockery of "health care is a right not a privilege." When you can't afford it, health care is a privilege, and increasingly, a luxury. To avoid expensive fees the patient will often vastly underestimate the degree of his illness. He thus will delay going to the doctor until it is often too late. Roadblocks to the receiving of health services, namely, high fees, the invisibility or inaccessibility, or both, of health services, all serve to prolong or delay the patient's appearance at the doctor's office, clinic, or hospital. This delay often accounts for tens of thousands of preventable deaths each year. Thus, fees of almost any sort serve to delay treatment, increase the degree of the disease, and speed up the arrival of death. Fees are a health hazard.

To argue that fees are needed to keep away the hordes of "hypochondriacs" fails to acknowledge that even these people, at a minimum, need emotional support—a very important job for the MD.

Fees serve as a barrier to health care, even if it's only a psychological barrier. They lower the *demand* for health care, as opposed to the *need*. Thus, people in need of medical services often don't demand or request them. This artificial fee-barrier to demand allows the medical-industrial complex to maintain the chronic shortages in health facilities and manpower, while delaying government and consumer intervention. Yet when new facilities are constructed in a community, when health services become more visible and financially accessible, the demand for services rapidly increases. This suggests that because of fees and other hindrances to services, there has been a lessening of demands on the health system and a systematic underestimation of health needs. Thus, fees have vastly decreased the visibility of the health manpower crisis and the visibility of the crisis in the health system as a whole. Lessening the need for government or consumer intervention, or both, the fee barrier to demand preserves the profession's monopoly and autonomy.

Patients are intimidated and oppressed to the point where they are fearful of questioning the doctor's bills, let alone questioning them beforehand in order to choose the least

expensive doctor. It's interesting that the medical profession
which so values the "free enterprise" system of competition
completely discourages patients from shopping around for
greater services or lesser fees, as people do in a completely
free market. Doctors claim that their ethics place them above
the need for discussion about fees in a competitive, free, open
market. Yet, informed consent and simple, legal, contractual
law would seem to mandate the need for a full, open, publicly
accountable discussion of fees, where patients can truly choose
among competing doctors and health systems. Of course there
aren't enough doctors around anyway to allow competition,
and where there are doctors, a conspiracy of silence encourages price-fixing. This is why doctors are forbidden to place
the price of a routine examination or procedure in the news-
paper. While I do not wish to make a pitch for a free enterprise market, I mention the above only to note that physicians don't adhere to their stated public ideology and ethic of
a free and open, competitive market.

There is a true lack of free choice of a physician when most
people have access to only one or two doctors in their community. The patient feels medically blackmailed and fearful
of questioning anything about a doctor's or hospital's services
or fees. With this limited choice, the patient may be fearful
of an implied threat from the doctor or hospital not to treat
a dissatisfied, questioning, or complaining patient. Naturally,
the ideal characteristics of the doctor-patient relationship,
namely, equality and mutuality, cannot occur when there are
shortages in medical manpower and "patient power." Clearly,
it is not in the doctor's economic interest to respond to the
patient as an equal. Morality and ethics in the long run are
determined by power relationships, and if those relationships
aren't equal on a power level they won't be on a moral or

ethical level. At present the public has not been able to exert its power.

True freedom of choice over a physician is limited not only by manpower shortages, but also by people's pocketbooks. While the physician readily chooses his patients on the basis of their ability to pay, the patient has no hard data upon which to make a meaningful choice. Information about a physician's qualities are known, if at all, only by other physicians. If a doctor is guilty of any wrongdoing, a "conspiracy of silence" protects the profession and not the patient. Choice is further limited by maldistribution of physicians, as well as geographic inaccessibility.

As the "conspiracy of silence" prevents patients from making an informed choice of physicians, so does the prohibition against any form of advertising or publication, no matter how informative or relevant, although the AMA spends millions of dollars a year on public relations advertising. (The announced budget for the AMA fiscal year beginning December 1, 1970, was $35,762,754. This *excludes* budgets of AMA local affiliates, county and state medical societies. Virtually all this money is for lobbying and public relations.)

Ironically, yet consistently, "peer review" and the "conspiracy of silence" hide from the public the shortcomings of the profession, while it is considered professionally unethical for individual physicians to show off their skills. "Showing off" may encourage competition and accountability, and is thus frowned upon.

On the other hand, the profession uses the ethic of "freedom of choice" to fight different forms of health services, such as group practice. The AMA's rationalization says that if you are a subscriber to a prepaid group plan, you don't have your freedom to choose your own physician. While this is true to the extent that you don't have an unlimited choice, you at least have a more realistic choice than most patients, and in addition, the advantage of a comprehensive continuity of care more often found in group practices. Other advantages include some degree of professional team supervision and accountability, nonduplication of tests and procedures, since the group uses the same laboratory. A new member of the physician's group is used immediately to his full capacity, rather than waiting to build up a clientele, as occurs in solo practice. Group practice also allows staff time off for continuing education. The AMA's "freedom of choice" in essence doesn't give you the chance to choose a group practice over a solo one. Solo practice is a laissez faire market place where the patient, if he attempts to make a choice, will have to go shopping from one doctor to the next—running up more bills.

County and State medical societies have successfully lobbied in state legislatures and have made large financial contributions to legislators to insure that no rearrangement of any medical service such as group practice can occur without the approval of the local county medical society. One of the more effective methods developed by the AMA and its county affiliates for pressuring a legislator is for the AMA to contact the doctors of the major campaign contributors (usually industrial magnates) to the legislator's most recent election. These physicians then use the doctor-patient relationship to cajole and convince these contributors to pressure the legislator to vote in the "right" direction. This in turn is followed up by contacting the physician of the legislator. That physician will then attempt to persuade the legislator to vote "right"—usually far right.

Thus, county medical societies have been able legally, and otherwise, to block the formation of group practices. Group practices have been prevented by denying their physicians hospital-admitting privileges and the right to certification by specialty boards. Group practice has been fought by organized medicine because it tends to threaten their market control. It threatens the fee-for-service system, and thus unlimited fees, the lack of quality control in any form, and the addition of third parties which might demystify or expose the profession. The MD wishes to be supervised by no one. The medical profession is a licensed monopoly analogous to a public utility and thus should be publically accountable. Monopoly by definition means the competition has been eliminated—legally. In 1943 the United States Supreme Court agreed that the AMA was in criminal violation of antitrust laws in their attempt to prevent group practice and should thus be penalized.

Some people assume that since the physician has special privileges and high status, he will act with special responsibility. But that special responsibility is nothing more than noblesse oblige, an elitist role, inimical to the doctor-patient relationship ideal of a consultation between equals. High status is a result of high income, mystification, and professionalization. High status isn't compatible with equal status and quality care.

The angry patient who associates his inflated health bill with his physician's ostentatious manner of living has every right to feel that his illness has been exploited—it has. The setting of exorbitant fees, rather than embarrassing the profession, has been used by them to enhance the prestige and reputation of the profession. In a capitalistic society people like to feel they "get what they pay for" and that they want and "deserve nothing but the best"—especially when it comes to matters of one's health. Unfortunately, the size of a physician's fees has nothing to do with the quality of services he delivers, only more to do with the nerve he has in charging whatever the traffic will bear.

In no other profession or business, except for the military-industrial complex, is the supplier given such latitude to base his fees on his own estimate of the value of his services and the patient's ability or inability to pay. Quality and competence, fees and services, are judged, if at all, by the physician's peers, and not by his patients or the public. "Peer review" (i.e., review by other physicians) maintains professional un-accountability. At least twenty states have restrictive legislation, passed at the instigation of the profession, that gives the profession veto power over the implementation of group practice and prepayment programs under consumer sponsorship. The medical profession picks and chooses what parts of the free enterprise ideology and medical ethic it likes best and then uses them to protect and promote its profession and profits.

Rather than being free, the medical market is tightly controlled. There is no competition between physicians or hospitals or medical educational systems or ideologies or training programs. However, physicians could be well trained, in less time through an open-ended, career-ladder program, as opposed to the traditional twelve-year program. But the profession won't allow such experimentation or competition among various training programs. What changes do occur, occur as a result of compromises between the conservative and liberal wings of the profession and the medical-industrial complex.

The setting of fees is not a professional medical issue to be controlled by the profession, but an economic and political issue to be controlled by the paying public.

The clash between the professional image of idealism and its substance of capitalism is increasingly visible to the patient who can't locate a doctor, let alone afford one. While the profession's preoccupation with profit is understandable in a capitalistic society, it's no longer acceptable. If the economic system has created a nightmarish situation where the doctor's wealth comes before the people's health, then that system must be altered.

Weeding out a few, or even many doctors, or changing a few courses in medical school, or giving psychotherapy to every medical student and doctor won't change the profit-motivated system under which they are forced to practice, and within that practice, support that system under which quality, noncorrupt, nonvenal care and services cannot be inspired. Health care must be seen as a part of the social and economic system.

Medical technology helps to create a professional language of its own. The technical language serves to further mystify, obscure, and come between doctor-patient relationships. This decreases the likelihood of informed consent. The more technical the language used by the physician, the more he must expend time and money fully to inform his patient. Yet, if the patient can't understand the language, he is more likely to be dependent, passive, and thus medically ignorant.

A medical student, Michael Michaelson, writing in the *Nation,* reports: "When a student at my own school asked an anatomy professor why he used the expression 'pathogonomic of' instead of 'characteristic of,' he was told, 'Why son, the public might know what we were talking about.' He was being funny, but he was not kidding."

He went on: "In our hospital every patient, and not merely every poor or black patient, is a nigger. From the moment he is admitted, the patient is reduced to the status of a dependent, helpless, anonymous infant. His clothes and worldly goods are taken away, he is pushed about in a wheelchair, wrapped in a drab dressing gown, tucked into what resembles —certainly more than it does the adult bed of procreation and elective rest—a crib."

Patient ignorance can be profitable. In cases where a cooperative, fee-splitting arrangement has not been worked out, the physician may be motivated to offer a better prognosis to the patient than what is based on the medical findings. A good prognosis will discourage the patient from seeking medical advice from other physicians, thus allowing his current physician to keep him in the fold, returning on a regular basis, for treatment. Fear of losing face, as well as the patient, discourages the physician from referring the patient to a more competent doctor; he's more rewarded for referring a patient either not at all, or to a less competent doctor. In effect the physician takes advantage of the patient's medical ignorance.

Allowing only physicians, as opposed to other health professionals, to invade the privacy and apertures of the body and psyche enhances, in the patient's eyes, the physician's occult role as an authoritative and protective figure. Perhaps the relationship would be more objective, less occult and less mystical, if, say, nurses and other professionals were doing the history taking and physical examination. They can easily be trained to do so.

The result of professionalism, mystification, and patient dependency was demonstrated in a survey made a few years ago by Florida State University. In a random survey, people were asked what they looked for in choosing a physician.

Virtually none of the respondents mentioned the single most important criteria in choosing a physician—competence. This has resulted from a number of circumstances:

The profession has perpetuated the myth that a doctor licensed is a doctor qualified. This has been disproved too many fatal times. And the profession has promoted mysticism and patient dependency so that patients don't ask questions about the quality and quantity of care they receive.

To remain as autonomous as possible in order to charge maximally for minimal services, the profession has refused any third party, outside quality controls, with the rationalization that only physicians can judge the quality of other physicians. The profession's ethics are there to insure that only the members of the profession regulate themselves. Many professionals place the number of unethical physicians at a minimum of 10 per cent of the profession—that's close to thirty thousand doctors who might in turn be responsible for the care of twenty to thirty million Americans. One malpractice lawyer Melvin Belli, has said that as the result of malpractice suits, kickbacks, overreferrals, overprescribing, overhospitalizing and fee splitting in 1960, in the United States only 32 MD's were disciplined—out of 230,000 licensed at that time. Such are the results of "peer review" and "self-regulation." The AMA's own candid report on ethics was ordered to be hidden from public view—which it was, except for a few leaked copies. Such is the profession's interest in ethics and accountability, such is their reliability in cleaning up their own house. Only the consumer can do that, because it is in his self-interest to do so. Medical society grievance committees are there to serve the profession and not the patient. The only physicians ever penalized are narcotic addicts and MD's performing abortions. The addicts and abortionists harm the image of the profession, which is the major reason they are censured.

A good deal of information about the quality of health care can be ascertained by nonphysicians and patients, but it might require consumer control of the health system to produce this kind of accountability. The medical profession on its own is notoriously negligent about ridding its ranks of those who are incompetent or unethical. Below are some examples of some simple screening questions a patient might ask himself or herself in order to evaluate some aspects of a physician's performance or—how to give your doctor a checkup!

1. When you see a doctor for the first time for an examination, is *every* part of your body at one time or another in that exam, exposed and examined, including rectal exams?

2. Does your doctor or his nurse on your initial full examination inquire about allergic reactions to medications and other substances?

3. Does your doctor or his staff ask about your family members' disease history, e.g., has anybody in your immediate family had TB, cancer, diabetes, heart disease, high blood pressure, etc.?

4. Are you questioned about your own previous hospitalizations and operations? Does the physician make arrangements with you to gather your previous hospital records by having you sign a medical records release form?

5. If you are a woman patient, does the doctor or his assistant take a complete menstrual history and inquire about pregnancies, abortions, contraceptive techniques, and venereal disease?

6. If the physician recommends a lab test, procedure, or

a drug, does he explain fully its purpose, risks, and potential benefits?

7. Does the physician inquire about any "unusual" symptoms such as: "Do you bleed easily?" "Have you had any swollen areas or lumps?" "Do you tire easily?"

8. Is a complete personal and social history taken? Does the doctor have a picture of your life at home and on the job? Is he attuned to and does he ask questions about changes in your mood or appearance? If at the end of your initial full examination your physician has not yet asked you your age, start looking for another doctor.

9. Is a complete dietary history taken? Are questions asked about weight changes?

10. Will your physician show you your medical records and charts immediately upon your request?

11. Will your physician discuss with you, before the end of your visit, costs, billings, and financial arrangements?

12. Does your doctor answer all your questions in terms you understand and to your complete satisfaction?

Any physician not doing *all* of the above-mentioned items is not providing you with even minimal health care, in spite of its relative simplicity. The point is that whoever sets health policy ultimately determines quality and competence—a job doctors clearly shouldn't be doing.

Far too many people, however, have no doctor about whom to make a judgment of competence. An editorial in the AMA's *New Physician* has stated that ". . . a basic lack of understanding has led to sub-standard treatment of these patients (medically indigent) by the medical profession." While it's an understatement to note that the medically indigent have received substandard care, it is totally false to assume that the cause of that substandard care is due to a "lack of understanding" or a communication problem. The medical profession knows better than anyone why there are two classes of care, one for the relatively rich and one for everybody else. Any lack of understanding or communication that exists, exists for the patients who have been prevented from getting a clear picture of the economic and political realities of health care. More "understanding" on the part of the profession will help no one, except maybe the profession to bilk the people a little more efficiently. More understanding on the part of the people will help them demand and then *take* more and better services for themselves.

PART TWO

THE MEDICAL-INDUSTRIAL
COMPLEX

III

New Money for Medicine

In a sense there are two medical market places. In one, the patient relates to and contracts for the doctor or nurse or hospital, and there is a direct exchange of money in a relatively public transaction. The second market place is essentially a supramarket, not really very public or visible, where transactions occur only among the controllers of the medical system and those who set policy for it. It is above the public's purview, just as is the military-industrial complex. The consumer/community is the ultimate payer to both the military-industrial complex and the medical-industrial complex (MIC), and while in the conventional medical market place the transfer of money is visible, it is in the nonvisible arena that the MIC functions. It is here that the liberals will attempt to garner and control new billions of the public's money for the private use of the MIC.

The medical-industrial complex is not simply analogous to the military-industrial complex, but rather they are substantively alike and in many cases are controlled by the same people. Thus major defense contractors such as Lockheed

113

and the Rand Corporation are also major medical contractors and therefore influence policy in both complexes. For example, the Rand Corporation has provided much of the major systems analysis research used for counterinsurgency programs in Viet Nam. That same corporation also receives millions of dollars a year from New York City to "rationalize" its health system—another form of counterinsurgency.

It became apparent, certainly by the early thirties, that virtually no one could afford comprehensive or even general health care. It thus became increasingly necessary for governments to intrude themselves financially and otherwise onto the medical system. However, what pushed government intervention more than an inadequate and often nonexistent health system was the profession's lack of financial stability. The consumer, alone, could no longer (if indeed, he ever could) finance the medical profession and its associates.

In its "natural" (i.e., nongovernmental involvement) state, there is little profit to be made in the medical market place. Only a wealthy market created by government support can ensure a profitable income from illness for the medical-industrial complex. Since only the federal government had sufficient funds, state and local governments have become increasingly, though not yet completely, irrelevant in terms of insuring an adequate (adequate for profit) influx of money. Just as there is no real profit in the defense (really war) industry without two basic components, namely war and a federal government to purchase war goods and services; there is no real profit in the health (really illness) industry without two basic components, namely, illness and a federal government to purchase illness-related goods and services. From federal intervention, however, evolved a basic split between the conservatives of the medical profession and the liberals of the medical-industrial complex. The schism between the profession (the AMA) and the MIC represents the natural evolution of a capitalistic economy as it becomes more advanced technologically and imperialistically. To support the market for serious advances in both technology and imperialism required federal subsidization and "intervention."

To the old line, entrepreneurial, single-man business types of the AMA, the federal influx did indeed seem to be intervention. To the more advanced members of the corporately liberal medical-industrial complex, the influx was an absolute necessity. In effect the institutions and corporations of the medical-industrial complex have been willing to risk that the federal influx of money will not result in the federal control of these institutions and corporations. The medical-industrial complex has good reason to be optimistic about their prospects. They have the precedent set by the military-industrial complex, where the government not only avoided any form of control, but in fact did all in its power to insure corporate autonomy and profits, if not military-corporate control of the government.

The split over federal and third-party financing in the health arena was delineated by Eric Lessenger of New York University School of Medicine:

While the inadequacy of health care in America excellently illustrates the indifference of American capitalism to the masses of people, it does not explain it.

The struggle between the AMA and HEW about the appointment of Dr. John Knowles was not so much evidence of "disease within the medical calling," but rather of the transition of power which is occurring in medicine.

Medicine as a sector of the economy has lagged behind in its development (precisely because of the strength of the

AMA) and only now are we beginning to see the shift from the individual small entrepreneurs, represented by the AMA, to the monopoly capitalist, based in such institutions as the university medical centers and Blue Cross and represented by such individuals as Dr. Knowles and Dr. Roger O. Egeberg, the man who finally did get the HEW post.

To speak of Dr. Knowles as a better candidate than the AMA's antediluvian choice is to misunderstand the nature of American health economics. If Dr. Knowles is more "advanced or progressive" it is an advancement or progression only along the lines of capitalistic economic evolution, and not along the lines of insuring for the people a health system that is publicly accountable and accessible, single and free, comprehensive and consumer controlled. Dr. Knowles is part of the progressive wing of the capitalistic class. He is a corporate liberal, and as such is no more likely to resolve the contradiction of making profit from people's health needs than the AMA.

The AMA is still an important reactionary force, but as Lessenger points out: "socially responsible people should be aware of the danger of allying with the corporate liberals in order to defeat the AMA." Such a danger is real, for example, in the revival of the demand for comprehensive national health insurance, which is now being made by liberal forces led by groups such as the United Auto Workers' Union. While passage of this proposal would be a great defeat for the AMA (at least ideologically, if not economically, after the model of Medicare), it would in all probability be just a mechanism for keeping money flowing through presently established channels. It would not lower the cost, improve the quality, change the class-exploitive nature, rationalize the system in a socially responsive and responsible way, shift the emphasis from cure to prevention, or make any of the other badly needed changes in our health care system. It would only serve to consolidate the power of Blue Cross and the rest of the liberal corporate class of the medical-industrial complex.

In effect then, economic evolution has led to the coordinated and incorporated organization of medical resources, manpower, and facilities. Thus mechanisms, devices, and institutions such as medical insurance, group practices, medical centers, medical planning councils, and governmental agencies at all levels evolved into and became parts of the medical-industrial complex.

Who and what make up the medical-industrial complex? Quite simply, it's composed of liberal doctors, hospitals, university medical centers, hospital suppliers and contractors, drug and insurance companies, nursing homes and "think tanks," certain banks and financial institutions, as well as a number of the major defense contractors. Last, but far from least, are major governmental planning boards, agencies, and departments, including the Department of Defense.

The MIC functions similarly to a conglomerate of large corporations. Large corporations to be profitable must be able to expand their profits continuously, must be able to plan the accumulation, use, and promotion of their resources, manpower, capital, facilities, and materials, a decade or more into the future. To do so in the American system, these corporations must be able to make public policy—or at least to strongly influence policy decisions, which is what both the medical and the military-industrial complexes do.

The MIC and the military-industrial complex are united ideologically in that both the medical and defense systems are run for the primary purpose of insuring profits for both complexes. Everything else is coincidental or there to preserve an image of legitimization and an aura of service.

While in general the overall purpose of the medical system is to provide profits for the MIC, in particular the medical system embraces four major economic functional areas:

1. *Extraction.* In this case disease is used (i.e., "extracted" as "raw" material) to insure the maintenance and expansion of research and training institutions. Disease is also used for the creation of new industries and areas of diversification for those industries—in essence, to insure an expanding market for the MIC.

2. *Labor Maintenance.* Health care insures the maintenance of a relatively functioning labor source, necessary for the continuation of a profitable general economy. A former vice-president of Ford Motor Co. said that health care should be available to all workers, ". . . to keep them healthy and *productive"* (emphasis added).

3. *Incarceration, socialization and channelization.* Health care helps maintain a stable population and insures a stable economy. This function is carried out by psychiatric services, particularly community mental health centers, guidance centers, as well as nursing homes. The famous medical historian Dr. Henry Sigerist said: "The goal of medicine is *to keep man adjusted* to his environment as a *useful* member of society or to *re-adjust him."* (Italics mine). The May 17, 1969, *New York Times* reported that "Psychiatry aims at the systematic subordination of individual behavior to false social norms." Not surprisingly, the new head of New York City's Health Service Administration is a former counterinsurgency expert, having gained valuable experience in the United States State Department's Latin American Division.

4. *Luxury items.* These are for a special few and it amounts to the special care, services, and equipment received by and reserved for the privileged class, that is, private nurses, private medical "pavilions," and so forth.

The Student Health Organization noted that: "Capitalism bloomed during and because of the industrial revolution. Not surprisingly, then, many of its institutions resemble the industrial model. That is, a small group of people at the top determines policy, the industry creates the product, the product must be sold on the market, and people must consume the product. The model has survived for several centuries." However, the needs and changes in postwar capitalism demanded the corporate organization "of all social services. A sick person, conceived as human capital, is no better than a broken machine." In line with the economic requirements of capitalism "the health system was developed in tune with the industrial model. Consequently health facilities and services were made a saleable commodity." In the 1970's playing with people's lives for the sake of profit is no longer tolerable—if indeed it ever was.

The more government money is poured into the medical market place via the MIC the more the health system will behave precisely as any other industry in the general economic system. In fact, the medical system will be literally composed of and controlled by the same companies which have diversified into health areas or merged with health-related industries or which have related to health previously but are now buying into the more conventional business enterprises. The American medical system is rapidly becoming a part of the American business system—only this time the commodity may be your life. Some of the major firms moving into the health arena include Lockheed, Rand, Dupont, and Dow—all of whom have heavily profited from the influx of federal money into the defense industries. They now plan to diversify into, or merge with, health-related industries and thus leech off any profit from the federal financial influx into the health system and industry. Thus, manufacturers of plastics and disposables for the war machine, such as Dow, provide similar services for the medical machine. Electronics and engineering firms design new, exotic, expensive, and generally nonimplementable (for the general public) devices.

In addition to the diversification process is the mechanism of conglomeration. Thus, for example, pharmaceutical firms now increasingly use their resources to research and develop cosmetics.

The advent of both the federal influx of money and planning has allowed the health economy to "progress" toward diversification from two different directions:

First, because of the continued and growing influx of federal money, profit seekers have increasingly seen the health industry as a "growth industry"—as an area for new investments and developments. Thus we see established companies "spinning off" subsidiary health research and development, hospital supply, and nursing home enterprises.

On the other hand, with a possible increase in federal regulation and planning, increasingly regulated companies such as the drug industry look for new areas to insure profit maximization and thus to develop new lines such as sunlamps, sauna baths, and the like.

Finally, as the economy reaches new levels of complexity and sophistication as overt war no longer remains a viable and stable market entity, the search will be, and is already on, for new markets. The rapid increase in the aerospace industry is an example of this. However, both war and space industries have specific limitations, as well as engendering political opposition. On the other hand, the health market is virtually untapped. At least a half of the nation doesn't even begin to receive adequate health care. While the health arena has increasingly attracted expanding and diversifying industries, these industries have approached the health scene cautiously.

The technology and technically trained people that go into, and are involved with, industries tangentially related to health, such as the health-leisure industry, are a constant source of brain and technology drain from the conventional health system. These people are almost all publicly trained and yet work for private industry, having little beneficial impact on the health system. For example, we are spending more potential health dollars for permanent waves than for the training of health professionals. Research in shampoos and permanents requires years of training in the research of protein chemistry. (Hair is predominantly protein.) These professionals are virtually all trained at public expense and yet contribute little to public medical services.

This is a situation similar to the military-industrial complex, where physicists and chemists trained at public expense research and produce material for warfare and not welfare.

The research and computer specialists are doing nothing more than tying into, and hooking up with, an inhumane health system. The computer people have been spending more time, money, and research on developing systems of billing people than they have on health programs. Essentially they are doing nothing more than computerizing a rotten system: garbage in—garbage out.

Health technology companies enhance their advisory boards

with white-coated MD's, supported by expensive retainer fees. This is the new MD compared to the old-line entrepreneur. The research developed by these companies tends to look like that of the automotive industry—stylistically changed, substantively unchanged, and ultimately dangerous. This insidious practice has been profitable for the drug industry, patenting and profiting from minimally molecularly changed drugs, and fixed drug combinations. The industry has attempted to pass these off as substantively changed, viable alternatives. The fact is that research tends to be along lines of commodity interests, rather than consumer services.

Where is all this leading to? As has been pointed out, the rising tide of technology is rapidly increasing the disparity between the level and sophistication of technology and the quality of services delivered to masses of people. This growing disparity will call for more intensive demands for political intervention. With the increasing realization that whoever controls health care in this country literally has the power to determine life and death for millions of people, with the realization that the people who brought us the war in Viet Nam are the same people now vying for control of our health system, will come the demand for wresting that control from selfish corporate interests and placing it in the hands of the people.

American capitalism has an historic trend toward monopoly and concentration of wealth. There is no reason to believe that the MIC will be excluded from that process. And with that concentration and monopoly come greater profits and less accountability. It is these new conglomerates of the MIC that will increasingly determine national health policy and not the recipients of services, whose only role will be to finance the whole deal. Public accountability and the meet-

ing of public responsibility, needs, and services is about as
likely from the MIC as it is from the military-industrial complex. Not even physicians will have a serious role in determining health policy. The major profiteers of the MIC will,
when it comes to money and power, make the high-salaried
doctors of today look like small town punks. Our health system has evolved from a doctor-centered to a hospital-centered
system and now to an MIC-centered system.

Consumer groups are no longer the only force fighting for
government subsidized health care. The MIC is fighting
stronger and harder than the consumer groups, but with a
different purpose in mind. The consumers want better health,
the MIC wants bigger profits. These are hardly compatible
purposes or ends. Bigger profits mean an unending increase
in inflation of the health system. Even if government financed,
the money ultimately derives from the people, who can
hardly afford a never-ending inflationary system. Unless all
aspects of the health system, i.e., financing, delivery, and
policy setting are under community/consumer control, the
MIC will get their wish for an unregulated, highly and
publicly subsidized market for themselves, as in the defense
and aerospace industries. Government subsidized consumers
without consumer control mean government stabilized and
guaranteed markets and profits for the MIC. The government, rather than guaranteeing fees and profits, must guarantee the provision of services.

Government-financed markets also insure a greater degree
of predictability and thus allow for the MIC a greater degree
of planning and safe investing and ultimately greater profits.
The MIC will therefore oppose the AMA's opposition to
government "intervention." The AMA's solo practitioner
prescribes fewer drugs, uses less equipment, and fewer facili-

ties than does the corporate health and hospital center—the retail outlet of the medical-industrial complex. Thus the MIC often has little need or use for the AMA, which is often in a position to slow down the process of purchasing MIC goods and services. Because the solo physician is inefficient in terms of the multiple dispensing, purchasing, and utilization of MIC goods and services, the MIC will increasingly turn away from the doctor as head of the health team and replace him with one of the MIC's own administrators, or even one of their own machines.

To increase and systematize consumer contact and thus financial transactions in the face of vast doctor shortages, the MIC will increasingly advocate group practices heavily staffed with nonphysicians, namely, so-called paraprofessionals, who will probably outnumber and in some situations outrank the MD's and assume many of their responsibilities. This raises the likelihood of the formation of at least some superficial allies, e.g., the MIC and community groups seeking greater use of paraprofessionals to solve physician shortages in group/ clinic practice settings with funding federally subsidized.

Where the community will come into conflict with the MIC is over the priorities of the system, e.g., teaching and research where equipment is purchased for teaching and research, as favored by the MIC, versus service, as favored by the community. Other areas of contention may focus on the issue of decentralized, small facilities versus centralized large facilities. The large centralized facilities have greater use for, and are better able to afford, heavier equipment, computers, television monitoring devices, and so on. Computer and systems people will attempt to rationalize and coordinate not only the hospital but entire regional medical systems. What the small hospital cannot afford, larger hospitals and all the combined hospitals of a region can afford in the way of even more expensive and complicated computers and screening devices. Chemistry and pathology laboratories can often be centralized, unified, and pooled for a number of hospitals for nonemergency work where specimens are sent (mailed if necessary, as is already done for some tests) for evaluation. Such centralized labs can then purchase the heaviest, most complicated, and most expensive equipment and facilities—not yet even designed.

The framework of health care which the MIC would like to effect is one where there is a maximum degree of subsidization and systematization, coordination and computerization, regionalization and rationalization, integration and centralization, very much a duplication of the military-industrial complex. Such a framework will maximize the marketability of the medical-industrial complex's products. The MIC will increasingly attempt to set policies that insure the implementation of that framework, and its attempt to implement such policies will clash with the community's attempt to set priorities for health rather than profit.

The only immediate possibility of difficulty for the MIC is that systematization may produce a greater susceptibility to accountability. Up until now the MIC has been successful in determining the nation's health policies and its delivery system. For example, providing equipment which can be used only in hospitals and insurance which can be used only for hospital care gives the large, centralized hospital an edge over noninstitutional, outpatient, and preventive delivery modes. In terms of influencing governmental policy directly, the MIC, as an increasingly concentrated financial and power base, can join their industrial conglomerate brothers in an industry-wide confrontation with the relevant governmental agency, department, or legislative body.

The numbers of people setting national health policy are few and their relationships politically are incestuous. For example, a professor of medicine at a medical school may well be on the board of directors of a drug company and do consulting for a "think tank" contracted to a governmental agency that makes public policy on health care. President Nixon's task force on national medical insurance includes representatives of Blue Cross and Prudential Life Insurance, as well as other board members of both the military- and medical-industrial complexes. Only one consumer or community representative sits on that task force. In effect the policy makers for health care, when they consult, consult each other and are accountable only to each other. There is no competition of ideas or humanely oriented innovations in services. There is a constant conflict of interest among the providers of services, the insurers of those services, the manufacturers of equipment related to those services, and the governmental regulatory agencies which are supposed to police the medical-industrial complex and protect the public and who, instead, do just the opposite.

The MIC will attempt to eliminate the AMA from seriously competing for policy control. Physicians are too expensive for the MIC to afford and too arrogant and individualistic for the MIC to systematize and coordinate. The MIC will increasingly rely on their own manpower and machines. Thus one MIC corporation formed the Career Development Corporation (CDC) to train health personnel to carry out many of the physician's functions. The OEO (Office of Economic Opportunity) has funded numerous programs similar to this for the training of so-called paraprofessionals. If the federal government goes in for this in a big way, as the MIC might want, the CDC would benefit from government investment in this area and in their firm.

In terms of machines, even medical computer manufacturers compete with one another, not on the basis of quality, but on the basis of console design, planned obsolescence, and appealing packaging. The planned obsolescence, the confusing packaging, the meaningless changes in design are all literally health hazards, as they make it increasingly impossible for one to make rational choices about equipment, its need, its competitors, and its quality. One is left to the tender mercies of the MIC when one has a choice at all. More often than not, however, the choice is not in the hands of the public, but in the hands of agents of the MIC in their retail outlets in the hospital. Many doctors, rather than fight their increasing subservience to the MIC, take advantage of it to add to their mystique. Just as your doctor has said only he can properly choose a pill and its correct dosage, he is now saying the same about diagnostic equipment and computers. Thus the doctor and whoever else in the future might be delivering health care and services, including machines which are more controllable and predictable, are little more than agents or salesmen for the MIC.

As Robb Burlage points out: "Faced with this growing MIC, the public is still unarmed and helpless. There exists no public apparatus capable even of regulating the broadening health industry, monitoring quality and controlling prices, much less determining social priorities for spending. The Food and Drug Administration has proved inadequate even to the narrow task of checking drug quality. More federal money is desperately needed for health, but it will be wasted unless it brings with it mechanisms for controlling the health industry—controlling not just the technical quality of its product but the developmental programs and spending priorities through which it controls the shape of the health services delivery system."

THE MEDICAL-MILITARY-INDUSTRIAL COMPLEX?

Is the medical-industrial complex a part of the military-industrial complex? If not the same as or a part of it, the MIC certainly shows numerous parallels and similarities to the military-industrial complex. While both provide some services, the major service provided is to its owners. While one complex claims to defend peace, the other claims to promote health. Yet both engender considerable suffering and death. The profiteers in one are increasingly the same profiteers in the other. For example, below is a list of the officers and trustees of the Columbia-Presbyterian Medical Center. Columbia-Presbyterian is one of the world's most prestigious and outstanding medical centers. Look who runs it, determines its priorities, and sets its policies. This information was researched by Richard W. Clapp of Columbia University, College of Physicians and Surgeons.

The following men are officers and trustees of Columbia-Presbyterian Medical Center:

1. Cleo F. Craig: President Emeritus of the Medical Center: Past President of American Telephone and Telegraph (At&T), number six in Defense Dept. contracts.

2. Roger M. Blough: Past chairman of the board for U.S. Steel, number 60 in Defense Dept. contracts.

3. Lucius D. Clay: General, U.S. Army (ret.); led first fund-raising campaign for Radio-Free Europe (a CIA cover):

board member of General Motors, number 10 in Defense Dept. contracts.

4. Joseph A. Thomas: Board member Litton Industries, number 21 in Defense Dept. contracts.

5. Augustus C. Long: President of the Medical Center; Chairman of the Board of Texaco, number four in Defense Dept. contracts, as well as a major polluter.

6. Frederick R. Kappel: Past chairman of the board of AT&T (see above); board member of Standard Oil, major polluter and number 24 in Defense Dept. contracts; board member of Whirlpool, major contractor for antipersonnel projectiles.

7. James W. Walker: Brady Security and Realty Corp., board member. (Note: The Medical Center's real estate holdings, mostly in ghetto areas, increased from $2.8 million to $8.5 million between 1966 and 1968.)

8. Milton C. Mumford: Board member of Consolidated Edison, a major polluter; board member Equitable Life Assurance Co. (handles millions in health policies); a major advisor to the United States State Dept. on overseas business holdings.

9. John A. Hill: Chairman of the Board of Air Reduction Co., manufacturer of hospital supplies and anesthetic gases (conflict of interest? Also there were almost 10,000 anesthetic deaths last year in which the gas played at least some role).

10. Robert D. Murphy: Former Sec'y of Defense; Director, Morgan Guaranty Trust.

11. Cyrus R. Vance: Former Sec'y of the Army, former Deputy Sec'y of Defense.

This is by no means the complete list. Those names not mentioned, however, all hold positions in major financial institutions or defense manufacturing corporations or polluting industries. Whichever, the rulers of the military-industrial complex have readily become the rulers of the medical-industrial complex.

There's considerable institutional interchangeability within and between both complexes. For example, McGeorge Bundy goes from Harvard University to become State Department advisor on Viet Nam, to the Ford Foundation responsible for the funding of numerous health projects. As mentioned previously, the present head of New York City's Health Services Administration left his job as director of the A.I.D. counterinsurgency programs in Latin America, to direct counterinsurgency programs against insurgent Latin and black health consumers in New York City—thus providing a more visible linkage between the medical- and military-industrial complexes.

Lockheed and Raytheon, both major missile manufacturers, have branched out into making medical education films.

Budget underestimations, budget overruns, and inflation are common to both complexes. See for example any missile program or any Medicaid-Medicare budget.

If the MIC has their way, the federal government will be paying most of this nation's health bills rather than the health consumer directly, and not guaranteeing the provision of services to the consumer. By paying the service purveyor, the government places itself as guarantor between the purchaser of the services and the purveyor of the services, just as occurs with the military-industrial complex. In both cases, the government as middleman lowers the accountability and responsibility of both complexes. Both complexes find it easier to manipulate and control the government and its central-

ized agencies, than the diffuse, less systematized, general consumer population.

While both the Department of Defense and the Department of Health, Education, and Welfare are engaged in "professional" activities, namely medical and military activities,
they both nominally have "nonprofessionals" or civilians or
"laymen" as their departmental secretaries. However, the
nonprofessionals are not in control. For example, the AMA
and its powerful fellow lobbyists of the Pharmaceutical Manufacturers Association, the Tobacco Institute, and some insurance companies were able to veto HEW Secretary Finch's
choices for assistant secretary and Food and Drug Administration Commissioner, respectively, Doctors John Knowles
and John Adriani, in spite of the fact that both men are,
ironically, on numerous AMA advisory and executive committees.

What is important to note about the MIC's power, or the
AMA's power, or the military-industrial complex's legislative
and lobbying power is that it is not the power of an isolated
industry. What's good for the medical- or military-industrial
complex is often good for numerous other service and commodity industries such as auto, banking, and chemical industries. These other industries lend their political clout to
both complexes. When the MIC or the AMA contributes millions of dollars every year toward selected Congressmen's and
Senators' election campaigns, they don't simply purchase a
Congressman favorable to the MIC's point of view, but one
who is favorable to the business point of view in its most
general sense. Such a Congressman will not only have AMA
support, but major corporate support. His campaign will
have been aided not only by physicians, but also by major

defense and medical contractors, as well as by major polluters. The aligned physicians, medical-industrial complex,
military-industrial complex, and polluters are thus represented by the same politicians. Thus for the AMA or the
MIC to come out against industrially caused pollution or
war is to come out against some of its strongest allies.

Just to suggest how concrete the relationships are between,
say, the AMA and both war and pollution makers, listed below are a group of major defense contractors and polluters.
In each of these corporations the AMA, itself, has made a
substantial financial investment. And the list is a far from
complete one. Companies and dollars of AMA investment
were compiled by the professional journal *Medical Economics,* in the April 13, 1970, issue:

Defense contractor	Item manufactured	Market value of AMA investment, as of 12/31/69
Honeywell	antipersonnel weapons	$2,971,500
Dow Chemical	chemical and biological weapons	$2,072,475
Raytheon	missile components	$1,965,000
I.B.M.	computer components for missiles and planes	$3,047,220
General Tire & Rubber	antipersonnel weapons	$ 843,412
Fairchild Camera	antipersonnel weapons, proximity fuses	$2,782,500
Aluminium Co. of America	missile components	$1,781,250

Data on "item manufactured," listed above, is published in
Efficiency in Death by Harper and Row, prepared by the
Council on Economic Priorities.

Not only has the AMA an investment in war, pollution,
and alcoholism, but a reverse process is also true. For example, the Tobacco Institute, a public relations front for
the major tobacco industries, has given the AMA a $10 mil-
lion grant to do research on, of all things, cancer.

Polluting corporation	Pollutant	Market value of AMA investment, as of 12/31/69
Ford Motor	auto exhaust	$2,261,875
Texaco	auto and industrial fumes	$1,531,250
Universal Oil Products	auto and industrial fumes	$1,381,250
Big Three Industrial Gas	industrial fumes	$ 500,825
Houston Lighting and Power	fossil fuel products	$2,370,000

And just to add insult to injury, the AMA, which is pledged to fight alcoholism, has the following investments:

Distiller	Item manufactured	Market value of AMA investment, as of 12/31/69
Anheuser-Busch	alcoholic beverages	$2,250,000
Pabst Brewing	alcoholic beverages	$2,208,000

The medical profession itself has played a supporting role in the Viet Nam war. For example, [the respected spokesman] Dr. John Knowles, representing numerous medical organizations on the Viet Nam Medical Appraisal Team, reported after his visit to Viet Nam that there was "no justification for the undue emphasis which has been placed on civilian burns caused by napalm." He thus contradicted reports from the International Red Cross, Physicians for Social Responsibility, and the Committee of Responsibility. And so we find that Dr. Knowles, one of the medical-industrial complex's chief spokesmen, became an apologist for the military-industrial complex.

If Dr. Knowles and his Viet Nam Appraisal Team are unimpressed with the napalm victims in South Viet Nam, perhaps they might feel different about some of the medical atrocities inflicted by the military-industrial complex on its

own soldiers with the complicity of physicians. In effect, medicine is used as an instrument of war.

The following project report of the American Friends
Service Committee shows very clearly the interchangeability
of personnel, ideology, and skills between the MIC and the
military-industrial complex:

Biological weapons constitue less than 10% of the U.S. arsenal
of CBW (Chemical and Biological Warfare) agents, the rest being
chemical. Furthermore, at least part of this biological warfare
arsenal will not be covered in Nixon's germ-warfare ban because of a re-defining of biological toxins, which was one result of
U Thant's report to the U.N. General Assembly in July, 1969.
That report, compiled by chemical warfare experts from all over
the world, re-classified the non-reproductive toxins, which are
produced by living organisms, as chemical, rather than biological
agents.

It was discovered that the first chapter of the U.N. report which
included the changed definition was written by a team headed by
Dr. Ivan Bennett, Director of the New York University Medical
Center, Research Contract Director of the Chemical Corp., and
an advisor to the Army on epidemiology and pathology. His staff
included three Pentagon officials, and the first draft of Bennett's
chapter was written by the Army's CBW experts, according to
Representative Richard McCarthy (D–NY).

In a telephone conversation with Dr. Bennett he reported that
his staff, even while in Geneva working on negotiations of the
final draft, were in telephone contact with the Pentagon every
day.

Thus, far from being banned, as President Nixon implied, the
use of germs in warfare has merely been refined. We now produce
a chemical agent extracted from live germs to induce the disease
directly. This allows us to apply the disease to selected targets
rather than to rely on random infection. Botulin bullets, then,

could be effective assassination or counterinsurgency weapons which would need only to nick their victims to produce death by botulism, the disease induced by the powerful toxin. President Nixon has renounced the militarily unreliable part of the U.S. biological arsenal and has re-classified the useful part, as chemical substances.

In 1968 our medical system killed, according to former New York City Health Commissioner Dr. George James, fifteen thousand poor people in New York City alone because of inadequate or nonexistent medical care. When such figures are projected on a national basis, perhaps upwards of half a million people die annually and five million people die each decade because of inadequate or nonexistent care. When one recalls that Nazi concentration camps killed roughly eight million people in a seven-year period, compared with five million killed each decade in the United States, due to a lack of conventional health care, it is not difficult to be concerned about the medical, social, and political priorities of the United States. Calling the health system and profession a death system and death profession hardly seems rhetorical.

Obviously there must be some advantages for the medical-industrial complex for them to want to maintain a multi-class society and medical system. In the most general sense the medically indigent represent a repository of unmet, untapped, medical needs. They are thus, at a minimum, a potential and constant source of unmet demands on the medical system, inflating the costs of all services, and allowing the purveyors of the services virtually to set their own price. The higher the demand, the less the supply, the greater the price and profits. In specific instances medical indigency insures a pool of patients to be trained and experimented on by med-

ical students and interns. The unmet needs of the poor allow
medical centers to apply for poverty agency grants which
allow the medical center to collect a great deal of money in
return for providing a minimum amount of medical care.

Of course, there's a severe price to pay for this class system of treatment and it's the poor who pay for it with their
lives. Because of unequal and racist application of current
medical resources, people die unnecessarily. What resources
are available are diverted to maximize profits. As the past
director of the American College of Surgeons, Dr. Paul B.
Hawley said, "In medical care . . . the love of money is the
root of all evil." Thus deaths due to cancer alone could be
substantially reduced at the rate of a hundred thousand
deaths a year, according to medical researcher Selig Greenberg. Fred Cook reports that his research indicates that forty-
five thousand heart attack victims could be saved if adequate
staffing was available. Warren Boronson notes that each year
more people die of preventable diseases in this country than
were lost in battle through all of World War II. To reduce
these deaths would require outpatient screening services and
continuity of care with inpatient services. It would require
services which are geographically and financially accessible on
an equal-for-all basis. To reduce these deaths drastically would
not require a scientific breakthrough, but a political breakthrough.

At a less tragic level, the poorest 20 per cent of the population has never been to a dentist, in spite of the fact that
virtually all tooth removals are preventable. In spite of the
fact that tooth decay is the most common disease in the
United States and plays the causal role in numerous other
ailments, the 1960 per capita expenditure for dental care in
the United States was only twenty-five cents per year.

According to the United States Public Health Service, children of the financially lower half of the population see physicians half as often as their wealthier peers.

We have noted that just as society's resources are distributed along financial and class lines, medical care is also distributed along financial lines and along racial lines. Thus, the life expectancy for blacks is seven years less than whites. Infant mortality for blacks is twice that of whites. Many doctors have tried to minimize our country's poor standing in infant mortality rates (i.e., eighteenth in the world) by saying our criteria are different from, say Sweden, which has the best record. Dr. David Rutstein, a professor of medicine at Harvard University, states that the criteria are precisely the same in the United States as they are in Sweden: ". . . I believe that the Swedes can count dead babies as accurately as we can." Forty-thousand infants per year could be saved if our prenatal, maternal, and pediatrics care were equal to Sweden's. Racism itself is often a fatal disease. What's worse is that the quality, and certainly the accessibility, of care is worsening as the economy evolves to a system where power is more concentrated and prices more inflationary. Certainly our relative *increases* in infant mortality and *decreases* in life expectancy suggest this.

Rearranging the medical system and transfusing it with new funds will be of no avail as long as the medical profession and the medical-industrial complex are left in control.

GRANTSMANSHIP: THE RESEARCH RIP-OFF

A vast amount of man-power and material has been diverted from serving masses of people to carrying out research in diseases which are not easy to understand and difficult to

cure . . . But no attention is paid to the prevention and improved treatment of common diseases.

—Mao Tse Tung in a speech entitled *Instruction on Health
Work,* June 26, 1965.

Background

A combination of forces, then, has led to the development
of large corporately structured and organized urban and university medical centers, and a federal influx of money. The
continued survival and expansion of these centers and health-
related industries depend on an ever-increasing supply of
federal money. One way to insure a continued and advancing flow of federal money is through "grantsmanship." With
grantsmanship, an institution must develop new and "innovative" research projects and service techniques, in order
to insure not only grant renewal, but the accruing of new
grants. These grants are needed to maintain staff and facilities, but they have nothing to do with providing free, comprehensive services to a community. The self-aggrandizing
aspects of grantsmanship, moreover, lead to a further fragmentation of care and a multiplication of the classes of care
available, while they simultaneously decrease the accountability of those responsible for providing services.

Just as in the general corporate economy, where some companies are more expansionistic and aggressive than others, so
it is in the health arena. Thus we see a corporate economic
behavioral spectrum ranging from guarded isolationism to
aggressive expansionism. The isolationists seem to be represented by old-line patrician medical centers with heavy capital endowment from private sponsors. They were at least
previously supported by a rich patient clientele served by the

solo private practitioners and researchers affiliated with the medical center (e.g., Cornell University Medical Center, NYC). Such centers are not as dependent on, or as interested in, federal support—at least so far. As the inflationary spiral continues, private sources will dry up and then even isolationist medical centers will "progress," becoming more expansionistic. The already expansionistic medical centers, on the other hand, will continue to need more and more federal money, but have no intention of providing more and more relevant services which might improve the broad spectrum of health care.

Because of this hodge-podge of services, grants, and unaccountability, the health-planning movement evolved, in an attempt to "rationalize" the medical market place, the medical-industrial complex, and the grants and federal funding that were supporting them. However, such planning and administrative programs as the Regional Medical Program (RMP), the Comprehensive Health Planning Act (CHPA), and New York City's recent Hospital Corporation Act have, according to the Health Policy Advisory Center Bulletin, "serious congenital defects; both are based on the long-standing tenets of American health policy of voluntarism and elitism which add up to the naive hope that if you give the most respectable elements of the private sector enough rope, they will eventually knit together a rational health system."

Reorganization of American medicine through RMP, CHPA, and Hospital Corporations has, or will, clearly fail. But federal sanctioning of regionalization, incorporation, and planning has resulted in two major changes. First, planning has been elevated to the status of a new "science" (therefore only "qualified professionals" can do it). Previously, planning was not only considered unnecessary but was counter to the spirit of a "free" (i.e., entrepreneurial) society. Some may still look with apprehension on the 1984-ish vision of health planners actually using the "science" of planning as a basis for decision making. But there is little substance to this fear. The actual health planners (i.e., the medical-industrial complex) are not about to surrender any of their power to the new health-planning technicians. The real danger is that health planning as a science will become a new mask for the current elite health planners, shielding real decision making behind a fog of jargon and professionalism and very far from the public view.

According to the Health Policy Advisory Center (PAC), the federal sanction of regionalization and planning is another symptom of the decline of the entrepreneurial doctor-dominated forces in medicine and the rise of the new corporate managers (hospital directors, deans of medical schools, insurance and drug company, hospital supply, and research company executives). Health PAC notes that "RMP and CHPA have done little so far by way of direct subsidy, but they have provided a flutter of Federal flag-waving for the corporate consolidation efforts. But the more consolidated enterprises are no more rational for the delivery of health services than the fee-seeking solo practitioner. The corporate forces have their own narrow institutional priorities which seldom include the delivery of comprehensive personal health care to the patient. Both regionalization and planning have become tools, in the hands of these corporate forces for further mystification of the decision making process." RMP and CHPA have shown, and the Hospital Corporation Act will show, that within the medical-industrial complex there is an absolute vacuum of concern for improving health services for the people.

Research

The economic imperative for expanding markets has created the need for increasingly complex technology and the research associated with it. Where and how research is produced, its quality and its quantity, bear little, if any, relationship to meeting health needs, except coincidentally or peripherally in an attempt to legitimize the research. Most so-called spectacular advances or breakthroughs are more the result of public relations than the product of physicians' research.

As mentioned previously, the 1960–1970 decade was the period of greatest United States health research expenditure in history and yet produced the least results. This is so because the research done for the most part was irrelevant, theoretical, or inapplicable, or all three, to human beings and what relevant research was done was not implementable or will remain inaccessible for the masses of people, due to manpower and facility shortages and a general public medical indigency.

On the other hand, implementation of relatively simple technical innovations, such as adequate prenatal care, nutritional and sanitation services would lower mortality and morbidity rates far more than multiplying by a hundred the number of hospitals doing open-heart surgery, or other analogous and equally glamorous and infrequent procedures.

For the medical-industrial complex which builds research equipment and facilities, for the university medical centers which house it, and for the physicians who utilize it, there is far greater profit, as well as personal and institutional prestige, in the control and publishing of research and research manufacturing than there is in producing anything medically relevant and publicly accessible. There is often more profit in developing medical technology than there is in implementing it.

For example, there are in the United States 777 hospitals equipped to perform open-heart surgery. One-third of these hospitals have performed no open-heart surgery. An additional one-third do less than one such operation a month. Thus two-thirds of these hospitals must remain fully equipped and staffed and yet perform exceedingly few services. Not only is this arrangement expensive and wasteful, but it's also dangerous to the patient as well. The quality of care, on the rare occasions care is offered by these hospitals, is quite poor. The care is poor because only an open-heart surgical team constantly and almost daily at work can gain the necessary experience and practice, as well as remain in top operating form. Without a regular and full operating schedule the patient is exposed to the unnecessary risk of an inexperienced surgical team and will consequently suffer for it.

The business of hospitals is increasingly business and not health care. In effect hospitals have become a retail outlet for the MIC's products. With this in mind it's not surprising that the MIC and hospitals have so many institutions *equipped* to do open-heart surgery, but so few actually doing it. The real profits are in the equipment, more than in the services. At the same time the MIC would oppose nonhospital, outpatient, decentralized, preventive oriented services which would be too small to purchase or to house such expensive machinery as that necessary to do open-heart surgery, even though such decentralized services would undoubtedly save far more lives in the long run. This is not to say that many research institutes and physicians are not interested in making medical discoveries. What it does say is that

federal and foundation funding of research projects is so unaccountable, so full of conflicts of interests between the
funder and the recipients of the funds, that the vast majority
of funds are wasted on worthless projects, or projects geared
more toward enhancing institutional, departmental, or professional prestige, or developing projects which maximize
the profits of the manufacturers of research equipment.

It is simply too easy to be heavily rewarded for nearly
worthless research work. With a health system chronically
and fatally underfinanced, most research is a luxury, not only
in terms of the dollars spent on it, but also in terms of the
space, equipment, and highly paid and trained professional
personnel who are diverted from the more mundane, comprehensive, personal, family, and community health services.

In effect, money goes where money is. Numerous private
and public agencies have made it profitable and prestigious
for the medical-industrial complex to devote a good share of
its resources to research areas, thereby insuring less resources
for conventional health services. The increasing diversion of
resources toward research and away from services guarantees
increasing inflation for those health services, which is to the
profession's advantage. Thus diversion of scant medical resources and a concomitant inflation have more often than
not worsened the very health problems the research was supposedly attempting to solve.

The words "medical research" have become an open sesame
to the Federal Treasury, where money passes from the public
till to private hands. From a grant, the manufacturer gets
his equipment paid for, the university medical center gets
25 to 35 per cent overhead expenses, and the researcher much
of his salary, prestige, and publications. And of course the
more research done, the more the profession can remain un-

accountable, hiding behind a smokescreen of technological mystification. And in spite of this, even if a real breakthrough were made, given our limited health resources and their inaccessibility, such breakthroughs must remain only of academic interest at best, and a cruel joke at worst, since they are not likely to be implemented.

The more government money is unaccountably poured into the MIC, the more the health system will behave precisely as any other industry in the general economic system. In effect the American medical system is rapidly becoming part of the American business system. It is important to note that the federal financing of health and health research is insuring corporate control of the health system and not consumer/community control. The federal money is *not* providing for a socialist medical system, but a fascist one.

If a hospital begins to run out of money, it doesn't cut the inflated salaries of its senior research staff or decrease its purchase of fancy devices. Rather it eliminates, to whatever degree is financially necessary, services to the poor and medically indigent or lays off (or both) the lowest paid hospital workers and speeds up the work for the rest of them.

The excessive funding of many esoteric research projects has been rationalized by claiming that it is simply impossible to predict in advance which projects will produce lifesaving and life-serving discoveries. While this is true up to a point, what can be predicted with utmost certainty is that the continued diversion of resources toward research will render health care more and more unavailable, resulting in the needless deaths of thousands and cause undue suffering to hundreds of thousands every year.

Many medical schools, in order to keep their researchers, their laboratories, equipment, staff, and resources at the medical center, have had to drain money allocated for patient services in order to put it into research, so as to attract more money and more research. Medical school teaching programs have increasingly emphasized research rather than service in order to utilize and maintain research resources. Hence medical journals are now brimming with reports of irrelevant research projects. In university medical centers, as in universities in general, the warning "publish or perish" is listened to by medical academicians whose salary and prestige are determined by the number of their publications. In an attempt to publish and prosper through research, thirteen thousand different medical journals are currently published. What is produced by new research isn't so much a new discovery, as it is a new article and eventually a new journal.

As in the general economic life of our society, public relations and promotion play key roles in medical research. However, if someone at Ivory Tower University Medical Center has a disastrous result in his research project, one never hears of it. To make such information public opens the possibility that grants will be taken away, research staff laid off, and equipment not bought. On the other hand, "medical progress" is highly touted. However, what's newest is not always the best in medicine, any more than it is in any other area of corporate production. As Dr. Walter E. O'Donnell, an editor of *Medical Economics,* says: "What you hear and see about progress in medicine is often stage managed by PR men, press agents and medical journalists. The information . . . tends to be selective, overstated, and generally long on form and short on substance. The day of the researcher or clinician working quietly out of public view in a dingy lab or at the bedside or operating table is long gone. To put it bluntly, health is big business nowadays—

one of the nation's largest industries, in fact. With this new status come some of the basic corporate needs and drives, (as well as destructive excesses), the need for constant, widespread publicity; the need to be one up on your competitors in the public eye at all times; the need to keep developing new markets and new customers."

Medical centers are increasingly dependent on grants. As one medical reporter noted: "Bashfulness and modesty seldom open up pocketbooks. Hence health has to be merchandised in a way that would have made the watch dogs of doctors' ethics pop their eyeballs a few years ago." Now with more power and wealth shifting to the medical-industrial complex, the ethics committees of county medical societies can no longer be concerned about such niceties, even if they wanted to be.

This growing tendency merely underlines the need for more consumer control of research. Research findings must not be prematurely released, so that improperly tested drugs or treatments are put into circulation. Failures must be publicized as amply as successes, in an attempt to educate people about the priorities and politics of health.

Just as the cost of research is accentuated by the advertising and commercialism associated with it, so is the cost associated with planned obsolescence and useless frills, such as glossier buttons on a computer. To make matters worse, there is no or little incentive on the part of the medical center to be prudent or carefully evaluative of any purchases made with grant funds. Any cost overruns are simply charged to the grant, or a new grant is applied for. Unaccountable and indeed even unconscionable uses of grant money have gone for hospital space for, and construction of, the private practice offices of physicians and for hospital staff physicians' swimming pools. Numerous grants have allowed for the purchase of much, untried medical gadgetry, for which standards have not been set as to quality, efficiency, or safety, and yet these gadgets will be used by and on patients. These machines have the potential for producing far greater injuries and fatalities than might drugs, which are somewhat more, but still poorly, controlled and monitored.

While the above is exemplary of research funds being diverted from strictly research use, what about the research funds which are used only for research? Well, for example, we've spent millions "proving" that cigarette smoking is highly correlated with cancer, in spite of the fact that the *New England Journal of Medicine* notes that the first clinical report linking cigarette smoking to cancer was made in 1761. A lot of good it did us.

The solution to these problems is not that grants should be eliminated, but that they should be dispensed on a publicly accountable basis. Grants should serve human needs and priorities and not institutional prestige and profits. But the growing dependence on research funding emphasizes the relationship between the medical-industrial complex (MIC) and the military-industrial complex. An example of an increasingly closer relationship between the MIC and the military-industrial complex is the use of Defense Department-developed MACE in state hospitals to control recalcitrant patients. Not only are we increasingly dependent on the military's funding, but on their research as well.

Heart Transplants: The Rewards of Research

For glamour, heroism, high finance, and showmanship, no area of grantsmanship and research compares with heart transplantation. More money has or will be granted for this research than for virtually any other in medicine. Certainly more money has been spent on the public relations aspect of this procedure than in any other field of medicine. And yet no research has ever produced so few benefits, in spite of the fact that millions have been spent for hiring well-trained personnel and purchasing (from the medical-industrial complex) the most advanced and complex equipment and facilities. Never has so much produced so little—for the public who pays for almost all of it.

What is so special about heart transplant surgery? First of all the obvious answer is that it is a life and death procedure. Unfortunately, we have been led to believe, via public relations gimmickry, that the operation is indeed miraculous, technically feasible, and rewarding. There have been plenty of rewards so far but none for the patients—and we had better not hold our breath waiting for them.

Those who have survived the operation have existed in severe distress. As Dr. Michael De Bakey described his philosophy about heart transplants, "I want to prolong life, not death." Tragically, all the survivors are virtually only temporary survivors; the vast majority will die within a year or two at the most from the time of their operation, and all will suffer false hopes and severe debilitation until the time of their death.

How can one be so sure of a virtual 100 per cent failure rate? Simply that the basic research in tissue rejection has never been done, and until it is, virtually all heart transplant recipients will die fairly shortly after the operation.

Why then have these surgical procedures been undertaken prematurely? Three rationalizations have been offered and all three have been strongly criticized by Dr. Dwight E.

Harken, past president of the American College of Cardiology and professor of surgery at Harvard. The rationalizations and their critiques follow:

1. "Heart transplants are therapeutic."

Heart transplants are *not* therapeutic. Virtually all patients die in a short time. Those who live up to a year live such physically disabled lives that it's difficult to conceive of that as living.

2. "Heart transplants are *experimental*."

If they are experimental, what is the experiment for? If it is to learn about tissue rejection, we can learn much better on the kidney than on the heart.

3. "The patients would have died anyway, so they lost nothing."

Dr. Harken reports that numerous patients have been referred to him for transplants, even though the medical treatment of their heart was doing fine. Thus, if these patients were to be operated on (as undoubtedly other medically stabilized and viable patients were) and receive a transplant, their life would have been considerably shortened.

Even Dr. Christian Barnard agrees that ". . . rejection of the donor organ cannot be prevented." Well, if heart transplantation isn't being done for therapeutic or experimental reasons, just what is it being done for? Grantsmanship rears its ugly head.

Hospitals, contrary to some sophisticated beliefs, do not grow randomly; they grow according to the direction which maximizes institutional profit, prestige, and prerogative and not in the direction of maximized services, except when large grants and funds can be siphoned off from those services for inflated salaries, prestigious construction, and purchase

of fancy equipment. Numerous institutions have rushed head-
long into this dubious surgical procedure in order to get in
on the ground floor of a swelling windfall.

Not only do the heart recipients not benefit, but the manpower, facility, and resources drained from other services
cause conventional services and their recipients to suffer as
well.

To make matters worse is the fact that the heart recipients,
and the patients who suffer a decline in conventional services
because of misplaced resources, are not the only victims of
this procedure. As Dr. Eliot Corday, another past president
of the American College of Cardiology, points out, there is
a double standard in the definition of death. That is, there
is a definition of death for the heart donor (80 per cent of
whom so far have been black) and a different definition of
death for the general population (85 per cent of whom have
been white). Such differences in the definition of death, according to Dr. Corday, leave the profession open to charges
of homicide or body robbing.

A white person in the general population is considered
dead when he has no heart beat *and* no respiration *and* no
brain waves. But the black man will be declared dead and
considered an acceptable donor even ". . . *while spontaneous
respiration is still present*" in him. This seems to imply that
heart surgeons alter their definition of death to suit their
grantsmanship priorities.

For attorneys Houts and Hunts, experts in medical juris-
prudence writing in the *Medical Tribune* of April 6, 1970,
as long as any heart beat *or* respiration is still present, death
has not occurred. This is precisely the commonly accepted
definition of death that heart transplanters have *not* adhered
to. They have not adhered to the common definition of death

because that would require the transplanting of a damaged heart, which, of course, would not be worthy of transplantation. Therefore, the heart surgeon is left with the dilemma of waiting until someone is legally dead and thus transplanting an already damaged heart, making the operation more worthless than it already is, or he can remove the heart from a patient who is at least legally alive. Since the vast majority of transplanters have chosen the latter, it suggests that institutional and professional greed may have led to nearly murderous acts.

The failure to do the initial, adequate research in tissue rejection, the failure to investigate the use of artificial mechanical hearts instead of human hearts, thereby avoiding two standards of death (as well as recognizing the fact that the number of potential donors a year is only around twenty thousand, whereas the needs of recipients would be over a hundred thousand a year, and thus only artificial hearts have the potential for meeting the full demands of the population), the complicity of major university medical centers, governmental agencies, and indeed much of the medical-industrial complex raises serious questions as to the real purposes of our health system.

EXPANSIONISM: ILLNESS, INC.

Hospitals: Physicians' Factories

Medicine is probably the only business where a factory for that business is provided at public expense. In effect, communities and their governments have pooled their resources to furnish the equipment and facilities for the physician-businessman. Hospitals are unique institutions. Physicians receive free of charge a capital investment of well over a

$100,000 per physician in hospital facilities, technology, and services.

The organization of medical care into hospitals, as opposed to isolated doctors' offices, simply represents a higher form of an advancing corporate economy, though hardly a more benevolent economy. Businesses assume corporate forms because such structures allow for greater efficiency and profit, though not necessarily greater services. The same holds true for medical care. In hospitals patients are concentrated in a small geographical area, adjacent to equipment, services, and the personnel to carry out the doctor's orders. The physician, because of the corporate organization of the hospital and his control of its technology and services, can see and care for larger numbers of patients than he could in an office or home visit. The increase in technology and organization of the hospital saves the doctor countless hours and needless labor. The physician, however, rather than passing on these savings to his patients, has used this new technology and organization as a rationalization for higher fees.

More importantly, hospitals and corporations exist to serve themselves, to enhance not only institutional prestige and profits but also the personal careers of its rulers. Hospitals compete with one another for grants, equipment, personnel, and the prestige and profits needed to obtain them. Competition among hospitals breeds duplication and inflation. For example, as mentioned previously, Senator Abraham Ribicoff (former HEW Secretary) reports that of the 777 United States hospitals equipped to perform open-heart surgery, one-third performed no operations. An additional one-third did less than one operation a month.

Along these same lines are the hyperbaric chambers (high-pressure chambers for increasing oxygenation pressure in the body) purchased and run by a number of hospitals for a cost approaching half a million dollars each. Not only is this treatment of dubious value, but the money could have been used for more mundane family services. But given an opportunity, the hospital will opt out for glamour and prestige. That's where and how the MIC makes its money. What expenses aren't paid for out of grants are paid for unquestioningly by Blue Cross. Board members of Blue Cross are made up predominantly of hospital administrators and other members of the MIC. Thus, Blue Cross simply funnels (or more aptly, shovels) the money into the hospital. The hospital in turn pays the MIC manufacturers for the new equipment. A major conflict of interest is often involved when the equipment manufacturer is also a member of the board of trustees of the hospital, while other trustees are on the board of directors of the Blue Cross system. Blue Cross reimburses the hospital whatever the hospital considers to be "reasonable costs." The situation has gotten so out of hand that in states such as Pennsylvania the state's insurance commissioner has ordered that Blue Cross cancel all its contracts with hospitals and negotiate new ones in which Blue Cross no longer reimburses hospitals for costs of no direct benefit to patients. Blue Cross was also ordered to stop charging patients for publicity, lobbying expenses, and expensive furnishings in administrators' offices.

What Blue Cross and grantsmanship haven't been able to fund, Medicaid has, making the illness industries virtually recession proof. Some of the newly proposed plans for national health insurance will make such a recession in these industries even less likely, as funding and administration will remain in the hands of Blue Cross and Medicaid—which is administered by Blue Cross. These plans, however, will not make more likely increased and improved health services.

Government expenditures on aerospace and defense research have produced an abundance of new, but not necessarily relevant, technology. The defense and aerospace industries have used, as one of their rationalizations in their appeal for more government expenditure in this area of research and development, the claim that this new technology will be applicable in medical areas and will thus enhance and save many lives. In an attempt to make this a self-fulfilling prophecy and to take advantage of a recession-proof, Medicaid-financed medical system, defense and aerospace industries, the mainstays of the military-industrial complex, are now developing expensive equipment and becoming a part of the medical-industrial complex. Unfortunately, these new entries in the race for the medical dollar have produced little or no improvement in health. Rather, through their encouragement of large, centralized facilities to purchase and house their equipment, they have inflated the cost of health.

To hide the scandalous expenses being added to hospital costs for nonpriority needs, hospitals have hired public relations experts to give the hospital a better image and to gloss over shortcomings in services. The salary of the PR man is often twenty to thirty thousand dollars a year. Hospitals, rather than being primarily health service providers, have become commercial outlets for their boards of directors and the MIC—who are often indistinguishable from one another. These boards and the MIC, along with physicians and their professional organization, set health policy for profit and prestige and not service and health. The new health-insurance legislation proposed in Congress would in no way seriously interfere with their continuing to set policy in a "business as usual fashion," which is precisely why so many of them are willing to go out on a limb and support that legislation. Much of the proposed legislation provides a new and sound fiscal base for them to operate from and leaves the MIC still in the driver's seat.

Banking and similar financial institutions are increasingly playing a role in determining health policy and priorities. First of all many prominent bankers and financers are hospital trustees. As the health crises expand more and more, many hospitals come closer to financial collapse. But let us be clear about this: the hospital as an institution is near financial collapse, as opposed to the men making money from it. Hospitals can be nonprofit institutions and still make plenty of profits for the people running them.

Hospitals increasingly borrow from banks to stay afloat. The banks borrowed from are represented on the hospital's board of trustees. The trustee in turn determines the interest of the loan, invariably favorable to the bank. Many New York City hospitals are paying, in interest alone, over a million dollars per hospital per year. Nonprofit hospitals, which nevertheless make money "in excess of expenditures," place that "excess" money in the banks represented by its trustees. Thus, profit or no profit, banks stand to gain from their connections with, and manipulation of, hospitals and their health policy. The costs of that connection and manipulation are added ultimately to the patient's bill.

Affiliation and Expansion

Hospitals, as is true for other corporations and the military-industrial complex, have a built-in impetus toward expansion. The impetus is built in by the medical-industrial complex which not only needs expanding markets and outlets for its products, but which is also increasingly in control of hospital and health policy. One method of hospital expansion is an "affiliation" mechanism. Such mechanisms are most common in metropolitan areas but now are appearing in suburban ones as well. A voluntary hospital (private, in spite of the fact that 90 per cent of their operating budgets are publicly funded, nonprofit) "affiliates" with a municipal, public charity hospital. The rationalization offered for this is that charity hospitals are poorly run and poorly staffed. The voluntary hospital makes then an offer to affiliate with the charity hospital to improve its administration and services, to improve its "management techniques."

The real reasons are different from the rationalizations. First of all the charity hospitals are in bad shape because they are severely underfinanced, in large part because whatever public hospital money is available goes to the so-called private voluntary hospital. To make matters worse, when the voluntary hospital assumes administrative control of the municipal hospital, it often transfers from the municipal hospital to the voluntary hospital important medical equipment. What equipment remains is increasingly utilized for the research and teaching priorities of the new administrators. The municipal charity hospital provides for the voluntary (usually a university-voluntary hospital) hospital tremendous patient resources for research and teaching. Charity patients in charity hospitals are forced to be research and teaching subjects for the new administration's staff. Poor patients who might have "sneaked" into the voluntary hospital prior to the affiliation are now excluded and dumped on the municipal hospital.

The research and teaching priorities of the new administration call for the development of specialty and subspecialty
clinics and wards, which tend to highly fragmentize services,
making comprehensive care an impossibility. The fragmentation and multiplication of overlapping services increase their
costs; but this needn't concern the new administration as it
is paid for by the city. The multiplication of services provides
additional sources of salaries for doctors from the voluntary
hospital who can now serve in the charity hospital as well.
As long as the voluntary hospital administers the public
charity hospital, the newly transferred doctors will get paid
full-time salaries even though they may not work in the city
hospital more than twenty hours a week, as is seen at Bellevue
and Kings County hospitals. Bellevue is affiliated with and
administered by New York University Medical Center; Kings
County Hospital by Downstate Medical Center.

With the city government as a financial base, but with the
private hospital in control, public money can be tapped for
the purchase of new fancy, but often irrelevant, equipment.
Because the new adminstrator's priorities are profits and prestige, gained primarily through research and teaching programs, outpatient and preventive services will be starved. In
effect affiliation is nothing short of colonization. The charity
hospital's resources, its raw materials, if you will, i.e., city
financing, publicly purchased equipment, and indigent patients, are usurped and refined by the voluntary hospital administration into a finished product of research and teaching
programs. In New York, state and city investigating teams
disclosed that voluntary hospitals were using affiliation money
for payroll padding, removal of equipment, and professional
absenteeism. In essence a public hospital is turned into a
private enclave.

Unfortunately, New York City is being sucked financially dry by its affiliation program. More and more public money is winding up in the private coffers of private hospitals, while services are cut back again and again at the municipal hospitals. Needless to say, the voluntary hospital predominantly services middle-class whites; the municipal hospital "provides" for the poor, blacks, and Puerto Ricans. What's occurring in the New York City affiliation programs is in all likelihood predictive of other metropolitan hospital systems. As New York's financial and hospital crisis worsens (and each crisis area contributes to the other), the city fathers are looking for a way out of this politically embarrassing quagmire. The solution they have come up with—or have been forced to accept—is the Hospital Corporation Plan. In essence the Corporation Plan entails the city's turning over to a corporation or authority all its eighteen municipal hospitals. The Corporation functions as a nonprofit authority, much as does a highway, bridge, tunnel, or transportation authority. The Corporation will then run the hospital system in a more "businesslike manner." Unfortunately, just as most highway or tunnel authorities have as their board members, members of the boards of contracting corporations, e.g., builders, bankers, and manufacturers, so will the Hospital Corporation have as members of its board, members of the medical-industrial complex, and thus be guilty of conflicts of interest.

The Corporation, aside from being financed by numerous governmental agencies, may sell bonds to raise money. This gives the Corporation a different constituency from its predecessor, the Hospital Department. At least nominally, the Hospital Department had as its constituency the general public. The Corporation will have as its major constituency bond holders and buyers. The only legal obligation of the

Corporation then is to pay regularly on its interest rates, even if this means slicing health services.

The formation of a Hospital Corporation is simply representative of the most advanced stage of monopoly capitalism in the health system. It makes the medical-industrial complex, which previously controlled only hospitals and corporations, the major public funding and regulatory agency for health in the city as well. That is, the Hospital Corporation represents an extremely high level of concentrated wealth and power. What happens with New York's Hospital Corporation should be closely watched by consumers in other cities as a harbinger of future health trends.

The MIC has been responsible for the continuing and expanding health crisis. At least in New York City, the crisis in large part has been exacerbated because of the hospital affiliation program. The Corporation plan, rather than punishing those guilty hospitals and the MIC, gives them new unprecedented and unaccountable authority.

While some hospitals expand by affiliating with other hospitals, some voluntary hospitals expend geographically, into the community which surrounds and increasingly confronts them. The word "community" is all too often a euphemism for ghetto. Hospitals in search of new space for research and teaching equipment and facilities expand into the area of least resistance—in all likelihood, the poorest and blackest area near the hospital. By the use of urban renewal legislation and public money, the critical housing shortages of our ghettos are worsened by the expansionistic priorities of our major medical centers. This is seen vividly in Columbia-Presbyterian's expansion into west Harlem for the development of a "super block." In parts of northern Manhattan, Columbia-Presbyterian now owns property from the Hudson to the Harlem rivers. A poor community is thus made poorer and more crowded, thereby increasing the likelihood of disease and the destruction of the social and political strength of the ghetto by fragmenting it further. Urban renewal becomes people removal. In an analogy to colonial imperialism, the hospital and its MIC associates usurp a ghetto resource (land) and "refine" it for profit. Increased hospital expansion, whether it be by an affiliation program or geographical expansion, means new outlets for drug companies, hospital suppliers, and contractors. Everybody has something to gain by hospital expansion—except the people.

IV

A People's Health Service

NATIONAL HEALTH INSURANCE

Well, where is all this taking us? It's clear we're going from one health crisis to the next. Health is more expensive and less accessible than ever, in spite of the promises of a glamorous technology. In an attempt to solve these crises, as well as to placate a population, not only sick about poor health care, but rising up angry against war, pollution, and poverty, numerous schemes have been suggested. All of these schemes and plans are, in one form or another, a national health insurance.

The idea of national health insurance is not new. The German autocrat Otto Von Bismarck in an attempt "to unify the nation" during a war, offered a national health insurance plan with his own particular brand of Prussian liberalism. Needless to say it didn't have its desired effect.

In 1966, President Johnson escalated the war in Viet Nam and at the same time signed the Medicaid legislation. Needless to say it didn't produce "the light at the end of the tunnel" or better health care, as can be seen from the chart below.

MEDICAID IN NEW YORK CITY

	Before Medicaid (1966)	After Medicaid (1970–71)
Eligibility for free care (upper income for a family of 4)	about $5,200, was to be raised to $5,700 in 1966	$4,500
Charge for a clinic visit (municipal hospitals)	0	$2–$32
Charge for a day in a hospital (doctor's fees are extra for private hospitals)	about $50	about $125
City tax money for municipal hospitals	$192 million (72% of the total city hospital budget)	$264 million (45% of the total city hospital budget)
City tax money for private providers	$60 million	$180 million

In New York City, for example, one can see that Medicaid has clearly failed. Those who benefited were private physicians, private hospitals, and the MIC behind them, and not patients. Physicians' fees, which prior to Medicaid had been increasing at the rate of 3 per cent a year, are now increasing at the rate of 6 per cent a year following the implementation of Medicaid, according to the White House Report on Health Care Needs (July 1969). A 1970 *New York Times* survey indicated that some doctors were charging up to four times normal fees for Medicaid patients. A United States Treasury official recently told Congress that "more than one doctor out of every three who has received substantial income from treating patients under the Medicaid programs appears to be cheating. . . ."

The failure of Medicaid is important to note. It has many

of the features of the varying national health insurance legislation now before Congress. A summary of these plans is charted in Appendix B.

What are the features fatal to the Medicaid program which are present in all the current national health insurance proposals? First and foremost is what the AMA calls "peer review." The "peers" referred to are the peers of the AMA, namely, the doctors of the AMA. "Peer review" of national health insurance is a euphemism for doctor control of the health system. "Peer review," or at least a doctors' veto power, will allow physicians and hospitals to charge what they wish and in any manner that they wish. While some plans give doctors a little less leeway than others, there simply is no *mandated* method proposed which places a serious limit on doctor and hospital fees, and thus no way to limit two of the major causes of the inflating costs of health. What limits are placed on doctors' fees can easily be compensated for by seeing more patients and spending less time with each of them. And we have already seen that limits on hospital charges will be met by holding workers' wages and cutting services rather than eliminating extraneous research equipment and facilities. Or worse, if a hospital or a doctor is prepaid, the hospital or the doctor may attempt to limit services, no matter how needed they may be. Nor is there any serious attempt to eliminate the fee-for-service payment procedure with all its pitfalls of assembly-line practice and overutilization of services and facilities.

The new national health insurance plans, like Medicaid, simply provide a new stabilized financial base from which the medical-industrial complex will reap new profits. What the doctors don't control, the MIC will. And there is no reason to assume that the MIC will encourage more accessible, decentralized, and preventive oriented services. Nothing in this legislation insures an adequate, accessible, and appropriate supply of personnel, equipment, or facilities, without which there is a relative overdemand and more inflation.

With regard to these plans there is no indication that a doctor will work in the ghetto as opposed to the suburbs, that hospitals will provide for conventional, comprehensive, and chronic family services and not heart transplantation research, that clinics will deal with addiction, venereal disease, abortion on demand, and arthritis and not obscure and rare diseases, that care would be continuous and not fragmented. Just to mention an example of what fragmented care is: Between March and November of 1969 a black infant girl was treated forty-four times at Bellevue Hospital, a New York City municipal hospital, during the first nine months of her life and never saw the same doctor twice. And just to mention an example of inappropriate care, in a case which is far from unusual: An elderly man was given tests costing four thousand dollars that showed he had a serious heart condition. He was then discharged and sent home to climb, many times a day, the five flights to his apartment. At the other extreme of inappropriate care and misplaced priorities is the Dean of Columbia University's medical school jetting to Europe to treat Portuguese dictator Salazar for a stroke when most of Harlem's stroke victims are considered "inadequate research and training material" to merit admission to the university's Columbia-Presbyterian Medical Center.

None of the issues broached by the above examples will be dealt with by the new insurance plans because ultimately they are not health insurance, but sickness insurance. Rather, the MIC will continue its business-as-usual posture, paying attention to centralized, unaccessible, and inappropriate facilities, and the purchasing of complex and expensive machinery. Probably the most revealing statement about the national health insurance plans was made by the AMA. The AMA believed its own insurance plan had an advantage over the other plans because ". . . it would have the benefit of *stopping* the government *from providing* mass health care services" (emphasis added). It seems apparent from the above that the purpose, or at the very least, the result of all the plans is to guarantee payment to the provider, namely physicians, hospitals, and the MIC, and not service to the patients.

COMMUNITY CONTROL OF COMMUNITY HEALTH

Well, what are some alternatives to the existing plans and proposals for national health insurance? As an example, a number of community organizations in New York City are making demands for just such an alternative. The demands are being made *now* by the recipients of the health services, that is the health consumer, and as such serve as a model for community control.

This discussion centers on the demands being made by a community on the metropolitan health system in New York City. While the community making these demands (East Harlem) is not representative demographically of a cross section of American communities, these demands, nevertheless, are in many ways relevant to all communities, whether they be metropolitan ghettos or middle-class suburbs.

In effect, these demands call for a total restructuring of the health system and are not simply a demand for more money. The first demand the community made was for total self-determination of all health facilities and services in East Harlem, including community control of licensing and ac-

creditation of hospitals and medical schools, by an incorporated community-worker governing board. This meant that
ultimate policy-making decisions for all health care in East
Harlem would be made by the recipients of the services
through their directly elected representatives and by the
workers in the institutions providing health care. The community's definition of a health worker is anybody providing
a service relevant to health, whether it be the chief physician
of a particular service or the janitor who cleans up afterward.
The physician and the janitor would be viewed as equals in
policy-making decisions, when those decisions affected working conditions. While nonphysicians would have ultimate
policy control, this is not to be construed as having control
of the direct patient-care setting, where examination and
treatment are ongoing. That is, the community is not interested in telling a physician, for example, which antibiotic
to use for which infection.

What are some of the major implications of community
and consumer policy control of the health system? According
to the community people involved in the community fight for
community control of health services, the consumer would
respond in a self-interested way and attempt to maximize
direct and accessible personal and family services. This would
be his first priority. Of less concern to him would be training
programs, whether they be training programs for doctors,
nurses, or aides. Trainees cannot provide for the health consumer maximal quality care and even an aura of experimentation accompanies their training, as seen in the medical
students who are often given considerable medical responsibility in city charity hospitals.

An absolute anathema to many community-consumer
groups is research programs. It is clear to the consumer that

these programs rarely have any direct relevance to him. The unfortunate fact of life is that few research programs have an even indirect relevance to most health consumers. The above would tend to suggest that any health service controlled by a community-worker board would clearly de-emphasize, and perhaps eliminate in some cases, training and research programs.

What training and research might be deemed appropriate would be passed on and evaluated by the community involved. The burdens and rewards of training and research programs would have to be divided more equitably than they are. Community control would insure that one segment of the population wasn't more trained on and researched on than any other.

Since presumably and hopefully policy-making powers would be distributed equally and equitably throughout the community, equal quality care for all would be demanded. That is, the health resources of the community would be distributed equally just as the policy power relationships would be distributed equally.

Essentially all the other demands follow from and relate to the first demand for community control. All the demands attempt to maximize the community's resources and to allocate them in the direction of direct primary services.

The second demand is for the removal of all city hall-appointed administrators and staff who work in any East Harlem health facility. The city-appointed workers should be replaced by people chosen from the community. This is the community's attempt to maximize the resources of all community institutions. One of the potential resources of the community is the utilization of health facilities as places of

employment for community residents. The community would
have three priorities and bases for job appointment:

1. If at all possible the job should be filled by a community resident.

2. The basis for rehiring those already at work at the community institution would be according to their on-the-job
performances and commitment to the community, as judged
by the community. It is felt that a worker from the community would have the greatest stake in the welfare of his community and would work accordingly.

3. Community residents who desire work, but are undertrained, should be given on-the-job, in-service training with
open-ended career-ladder and educational opportunities. Performance and commitment would be the basis for evaluation
and promotion. This type of training of community people
is probably the only type of training program this community will relate to, given the vast depths of its service needs
which must be met before training and research programs are
implemented.

The third demand was for an immediate end to construction in the community of buildings devoted to health until
the community board inspects and approves or authorizes
new plans. Community control of health facilities means
community control of the initial planning stages of those
facilities. One of the major university medical centers in New
York City has had the construction of its community mental
health center delayed for four years because the medical center administration did not clearly involve the community in
the initial planning stages, i.e., long before even architects
are hired, as is required by federal National Institute for
Mental Health legislation. Certainly the community is correct in noting that its power and options are severely limited

if they have to deal with an already completed health facility. The community may have preferred highly decentralized, multiple facilities, while the hospital or health facility planners may have preferred an ultramodern, multistoried glass and steel structure.

The next demand is for free, publicly supported health care for treatment and prevention, including extended care services, such as nursing, psychiatric, dental, and home care services, as well as free drugs and appliances, such as eyeglasses, wheelchairs, and so forth. Elimination of all fees for any service or item whatsoever was demanded. Funding would come from the federal government's general tax revenues, making the tax base as progressive as possible. That is, the poor would be paying the least and the richest, the most. All but one of the suggested national health insurance plans have a regressive tax base. Funding would go directly to the local community health council, which would then develop, implement, or negotiate for services.

As stated, even by the AMA, health care is no longer a privilege, but a right. If health care is a right then it must be readily accessible, and fees of any sort place a limitation on accessibility, even if in some cases it's only a psychological limitation of accessibility. It was also noted that in New York City, for example, 80 per cent of the population is medically indigent, if not by official New York State standards, then certainly by many health professionals' standards. The degree of medical indigency increases way beyond the 80 per cent mark when one wishes to include serious, comprehensive, preventive, and enhancing health programs, as demanded by the community. To require these services creates a situation of universal medical indigency, i.e., everybody is in need of some public subsidies for health care.

If health care is a right, then no part of health care should be denied. If none is denied then we cannot have a multiclass system of health care. If a relatively rich person is receiving better care than a poor person, then, for that poor person the best health care is a privilege and not a right. Now what kind of implication does equalization of health care services have? Certainly it means the elimination of charity wards, unless we are all on charity. It suggests that there will be attempts at redistribution, redefinition, individualization, and decentralization of services.

The demand for equality in health services and health resources is an expensive and explosive demand. Just to get some idea of the expenses of a health care system meeting the criteria of equality, let's look at a few small examples.

1. The first example is air pollution, a major cause of respiratory diseases in the United States. Equalized services also mean equalized preventive services. Since some parts of the country have only minimal amounts of air pollution, we would have to meet that standard of excellence, that is, have equal quality control of air pollution. The United States Public Health Service has estimated that it would cost an additional expenditure of $10 billion a year to control all forms of air pollution.

2. The second example is lead poisoning. Again, there is no significant lead poisoning in suburbs. To achieve equality we would have to eliminate all lead-poison filled dwellings. And this can only be done by boarding up and covering lead-painted walls. Estimated initial expenses in New York City alone, which has close to one million substandard lead-filled dwellings, is a minimum of $100 million a year for the next ten years.

3. As a third example: to meet the suggested ratio of one

practicing MD to five hundred potential patients means training a hundred and fifty to two hundred thousand more physicians. That means tripling the number of our medical schools, that is, creating two hundred new medical schools at $50–$100 million a school.

There are numerous other examples of health inequities and deficiencies, such as the need to double the number of practicing nurses, to quadruple the number of paraprofessionals, quadruple the number of community mental health centers, to multiply by a factor of ten the number of satellite health clinics, and on and on and on. It is relatively easy to work up a proposed federal expenditure of an additional $100 billion a year. It seems clear that to locate and reallocate an additional $100 billion a year would seriously tear at the fabric of our economic system.

The impact of such a program on our economic system was exposed with the passage of Medicaid, which in many ways was only a mild reform and yet threw nearly twenty states into near or actual bankruptcy, before the states cut back on their Medicaid allotments.

Next was a demand for total decentralization of health services, with the appointment of block health officers responsible to the community-controlled board. There have been a few studies that suggest that maximization of decentralization of facilities in turn maximizes the visibility and accessibility of services. It also tends to maximize the health consciousness of the people in the vicinity of the facility. That is, people living near the facility become increasingly sophisticated about their health needs and will tend to utilize that facility earlier and more often. In essence, decentralized facilities have pulled a lot of sickness out of the woodwork. Families who had never related to conventional health services, families who died at home, suddenly began appearing at clinics for middle-class-type ailments, such as chest pain. Their sick-role behavior takes on middle-class characteristics. That is, when they feel pain they go to a doctor or clinic. All of which in a short time produces an overwhelming demand for the services because of an underestimation of the health needs of the community. The point is that, in planning services, chances are that if one uses conventional mortality and morbidity figures, one will grossly underestimate the potential demands placed on those services. Block health officers doing door-to-door surveys will uncover vast untapped areas of health needs. Health services located in areas of general usage, such as shopping centers, will allow those needs to be met more readily.

Most health surveys have been done by noncommunity people who made a one-shot visit to the community. Most people will not seriously relate their personal and private health needs to strangers, especially if they are clearly strangers from outside the community.

To maximize health coverage, to maximize decentralization, to maximize health services, we will have to multiply the number of health workers many, many times. It appears to be beyond our means to meet the majority of our health needs through physicians alone. Physicians are going to have to release many of their responsibilities and turn over many of their skills to nonphysicians. Clearly a vast army of paraprofessionals will be needed to provide health care that is of equal quality, care that is readily accessible and truly comprehensive. However, numerous community battles in New York City have suggested that the community and its workers will not be satisfied with simply transferring responsibilities without transferring a concomitant amount of authority, compensation, prestige, and privileges to the workers. The workers in and from the community, who control the community facility, will no longer accept the rationalization that the possession of advanced technical proficiency is a reason for advanced privileges, prerogatives, and compensation. If the community's demands do come to bear, it does suggest that there will be a deheirarchization of health-care teams. There is no inherent reason why a physician should be head of a health-care team. For example, in some cases he could very likely play a consultative role rather than a supervisory role.

As a Physicians' Forum pamphlet puts it: "The concept that control of health services should be in the hands of broadly representative community groups requires an altered role for the progressive physician. It means abdication of an elitest role in which physicians prescribe the structure of health services. It gives more explicit recognition that providers of health care are accorded the privilege to serve the community, by the community and thus are always accountable to it. The physician, in a community-controlled health service, is called upon to work cooperatively in a health team with consumer leadership, to respect the community's desire for self-determination and to pay greater heed to the economic, social and environmental influences on health. This new concept will enrich the role of the physician."

Next the community demanded door-to-door preventive health services, emphasizing environmental, addiction, and sanitation control, nutrition, maternal and child care, and senior citizen services. All of these services would attempt to meet needs not usually met by the vast majority of hospitals or services, yet needs which are of a crucial life and death nature. In the area of nutrition, few health services in the country have been as effective in combatting nutritional deficiencies as has an organization such as the Black Panthers. The Panthers distribute leaflets in their communities and personally speak to large numbers of people about malnutrition. White doctors have been assisting the Panthers, doing physical examinations and chemical screening tests for malnutrition. The examinations and the laboratory work are done right in the Panther office. Children found to be malnourished are then urged to come to the Panther breakfast program, where the children are politicized as well. As the Speaker of the California General Assembly, Jess Unruh, said, in 1969 the Panthers in California fed more children than did the state government. While it is clear that the Panthers uncovered a crucial health need and expoited it politically, another aspect of the Panther nutrition program is that the Panthers themselves have been taught to do the physical screening (examinations) and microhematocrit studies, thus demonstrating to the community the role of professional mystification in minimizing services to the community. By this is meant that licensing, educational qualifications, and so on have little to do with the ability to provide a needed relevant service, and that in fact the city cannot or will not provide these services.

When it comes to senior citizen care, many of the elderly are too debilitated to get to a hospital or to attempt to attend the various and fragmented speciality clinics. The structure of the conventional health system insures that these patients are "too sick to treat." The elderly are also the poorest and the most immobilized, often without phones or friends or sources of communication. Clearly highly decentralized *outreach* programs are required, and being demanded. That is, the health facility will look for and seek out patients and not the other way round.

Next, health education programs for all the people in the community were demanded. This calls for a new, responsive, and responsible role for a hospital or clinic administrator.

Traditionally, the hospital administrator has been the book-keeper, the gatekeeper, and the public relations man of the hospital. In general, he attempts to smooth things over, to be an expeditor, to run a tight ship and eliminate the visability of deficiencies and inefficiencies—all in the service of the board of trustees or the hospital commissioner or whoever is in charge. I saw a good example of this recently when I visited the state hospital in Poughkeepsie, New York. The hospital administrator was asked how much per capita per day was spent on food. At first, he didn't want to reveal that the figure was $.60 a day per person. When he finally confessed that figure, he hastened to assure me that it wasn't all that bad, and he hadn't seen a case of hospital malnutrition in years. There is a point to be made here: Who is the hospital administrator serving when he attempts to hide and minimize glaring deficiencies in service? Clearly he is not serving the interests of the community served by that hospital. If that hospital were community controlled, the community would demand that the hospital administrator publicly and explicitly state all deficiencies. They would make this demand for two reasons:

1. The explicitness of the problem best allows the problem to be dealt with in a publicly accountable and educative way;

2. The greater the visability of the problem, the greater the level of health consciousness instilled into the community.

The hospital administrator must help the community face

its health needs, which he can't do by smoothing over rough spots and doing public relations work. By raising the community's health consciousness by emphasizing deficiencies, it is easier for the community to determine the seriousness of its health needs.

Another aspect of the demand for health education programs is that they expose health problems such as sanitation, rats, poor housing, malnutrition, accidents, police brutality, pollution, and other forms of oppression. Certainly the people who formulated this demand had the World Health Organization's definition of health in mind; namely, that quality health services promote not simply the absence of disease, but rather enhance one's physical, mental, and social well-being.

Included among the demands for community education was the demand for a full explication to, and meeting of the "legal rights" of, patients. (For an example of an attempt to deal with this issue in the British National Health Service, see Appendix C.) Prof. E. V. Sparer, of the University of Pennsylvania's Law School, notes that in our country, for example, "almost totally unexplored are the legal remedies available to the indigent against health hazards in the environment which peculiarly affects the poor." Let us look at two examples. Migrant workers are exposed to health hazards by virtue of the excess use of pesticides. Do the federal standards established under the Federal Rodenticide, Fungicide, or Pesticide Act—for the violation of which there are criminal sanctions—allow for lawsuits by the victims? "What rights might be conferred upon poor people, who, because of patterns of zoning, etc., might be exposed to conditions of environmental pollution which violate federal standards or state compacts?"

From another perspective, one of the Constitution's expressed purposes was the desire to "insure domestic tranquillity" and "promote the general welfare." Implicit in these phrases are certain basic concepts of humanity and decency. One of these is the desire to insure that indigent, unemployable citizens will have at least the bare minimums required for existence, without which our expressed fundamental constitutional rights and liberties frequently cannot be exercised and therefore become meaningless. Medical treatment for a sick person is surely among the bare minimums required for existence. It is thus being suggested that an equal-protection assault on the crazy-quilt exclusions from medical benefits be initiated. Equal-protection cases would apply not only to exclusionary patterns in benefit programs, but to unequal methods and kinds of treatment within our health facilities. That is, there would be an attack on the dual system of care that exists in many hospitals, one for the rich and one for the poor. "Congress has made very clear its intent that medical and remedial care and services made available to recipients under Title XIX be of high quality and in no way inferior to that of the rest of the population."

Other areas of legal contention center on confidentiality and privacy. Even in some university medical centers, record room personnel are directed to disclose records to uniformed policemen upon their request.

Next was the demand that the community-worker board have total control of the budget allocations, overall medical policy, hiring, firing, salaries, construction, and health code enforcement. This demand is really the specifics of community control of health services. Included within the control of health codes are such things as building construction codes. That is, there is essentially a demand to control all aspects of policy that relate to the quality of human life, which is the definition of health.

Without control of budget allocations there is no community control. In many ways, no matter how willing the various bureaucracies might be to grant community control, it's still extremely difficult to achieve in practice. City, state, and federal governments ultimately control budget purse strings, and without the control of those strings, community control is highly limited. To limit the strictures on community control placed by the multiplicity of governments a community must relate to, community people are now demanding that there be only one governmental agency responsible for control of funding. Thus, if the community negotiated directly with the federal government for funding the community could eliminate much of the control of city, county, and state governments. With each and every community determining for itself its own individual state of care and systems of health, we might then be in a position to talk about a market place of competing ideas. Each community, in effect, becomes a social laboratory, each with its own needs and unique self-determined solutions.

SEIZURE OF SERVICES

The preceding section describes in a general way an alternative to existing and proposed health systems. It also implies that the strategy for achieving such an alternative will require a broadly based constituency, organized, educated and served by an indigenous leadership. The following is a case study (as well as a summary of the major issues discussed in this book) of an initial attempt by a community at bringing one of its health institutions under community control:

In New York City, in the first forty-nine days of 1970, 34 teenagers, including some twelve-year olds, in addition to 104 adults, died of heroin usage. This is an average of almost three deaths a day related to heroin usage. This mortality rate shows no sign of declining, but rather appears to be increasing. Heroin is now the leading cause of death among teenagers in New York City.

Eleven-year-olds have been arrested as drug pushers. The statistics, along with the visibility of the heroin drug problem, has been increasing astronomically. A recent unpublished study by the New York City Board of Education showed that there was, within a one-year period, a 500 to 700 per cent increase in the number of known teenage heroin addicts and in the number of suspected teenage heroin addicts. The rapidly rising death rate of addicts in general and of teenagers in particular emphasizes community-wide institutional failures to meet people's needs—not just by the health system, but by the entire human services network.

All the deaths have occurred in or on the periphery of the city's ghetto areas. St. Luke's Hospital is one block away from the Harlem ghetto. Though nominally a private hospital, 90 per cent of its operating money comes from governmental, i.e., public, agencies. In spite of years of pleading from and negotiations with the surrounding Harlem community, in spite of St. Luke's being a publicly funded hospital, it has remained publicly unaccountable to the community's overwhelming need for addiction services. Though it maintained no serious addiction program it did have, at least nominally, a Division of Community Psychiatry. The Division of Community Psychiatry is funded totally by public money and has satellite offices and staff. Documents from the Division reveal that the Division has contracted out its services to the city police department to engage in a "cooperative effort to . . . enable the police to function better. . . ." The major area of cooperation was "community relations," a euphemism for riot control.

Other documents revealed that the Division was about to engage in similar activities with the Defense Department's Department of the Army. Rather than being engaged in community service programs, the Division was engaged in counterinsurgency programs, with the ultimate use of psychiatry as a tool of repression and clearly of no benefit to the community. The police certainly did not need training from a psychiatrist to locate and arrest heroin-pushers, often operating on the doorsteps of the hospital. It is more than ironic that the part of the hospital which should be most responsive to community needs, the Division of Community Psychiatry, was the part of the hospital least interested in community needs. Even most of the professional staff within the hospital had never heard of the Division. This is not an attempt to single out St. Luke's as uniquely culpable; the situation is much worse than that elsewhere. Most hospitals do not even pretend to have a Division of Community Psychiatry—good, bad, or otherwise.

A disparate array of factors was involved in a rapidly developing crisis. Housing shortages were being exacerbated by land grabs for institutional expansion by the numerous hospitals and medical centers which surround, but poorly serve, the Harlem area. This deprives the poor of an already short supply of apartments and increases the rent for those which remain. This in turn makes the poor poorer and increases the likelihood of the correlates of poverty, such as heroin addiction. Increasingly funding of medical centers is dependent on grants for the implementation of innovative services. Drug addiction services bring in very little of this money and thus the services are nearly nonexistent. Addiction services also have minimal use for any form of technology and equipment, so that hospital suppliers and contractors can in no way profit from addiction services and thus they rarely pressure for implementation of these services. Addiction services are of no profitable relevance to insurance companies, as virtually only the poor are addicted to heroin and thus do not have and cannot afford insurance premiums—so no services. Drug companies also have nothing to gain from implementation of addiction services, as heroin withdrawal costs less than a dollar a person and therefore offers little area for profit. Even methadone maintenance is available cheaply. And as we have seen, these corporations—hospital suppliers and contractors, equipment manufacturers, drug and insurance companies, and other members of the medical-industrial complex—increasingly play a role in determining the programatic priorities of our health institutions, and addiction service is not one of those priorities. The hospital, on the other hand, requires an overwhelming and costly amount of bed space and professional staff to deal seriously with the heroin problem, and thus avoids it. Doctors are in general simply not trained to handle addiction services. Medical students aren't trained in addiction programs in large part because it has nothing to do with their future intended practices in the white upper-middle-class suburbs. Given the racial characteristics of a heroin addiction clientele and the racist nature of medical training, quality doctor-patient relationships would be at a premium. Overwhelmingly the problem of serious heroin addiction is confined almost exclusively to ghetto areas and thus seems to be a socioeconomic or politico-economic one and not a physiological one, and thus does not conform to traditional medical education ideology. Medical education emphasizes organic physiologic pathology and not politico-economic pathology, thereby insuring limited medical and professional interest. As reported on numerous occasions in *The New York Times* the local police either completely avoid arresting major pushers and suppliers or are complicit with and on the payroll of the Mafia, the major source of heroin in the ghetto. Thus the police, as well as the medical-industrial complex, have little or no stake in the implementation of addiction services or addiction removal.

On January 13, 1970, about fifty black, brown, and white members of the community, as well as physicians and other health workers from the Medical Liberation Front (myself included), invaded St. Luke's Hospital. We seized and occupied all the offices of the Division of Community Psychiatry, set up walk-in heroin detoxification and rehabilitation units and demanded that the hospital, as a publicly funded health institution, turn over 120 of its 800 beds to the community for community relevant services, i.e., addiction programs. The hospital up until this time had *selective* admission policies, where patients were admitted on the basis of their ability to pay or their usefulness in teaching and research projects. Therefore, in the last ten to fifteen years, the hospital turned away and chose not to select any patients with addiction problems.

Once in the hospital, Medical Liberation Front people quickly taught community people how to detoxify heroin addicts with thorazine. Methadone was not used because the community felt that methadone would simply replace one addictive drug for another. This teaching effort rapidly demystified the role of the physician, and transferred his skills directly to the community. From that point on, the only time doctors or nurses were needed was when severe vomiting occurred, in which case injections were used. In the three and a half days we held the building, a doctor or nurse was only needed once for the one severe case of vomiting.

Rehabilitation and education programs were carried on by a group called ABLE (Academy for Black and Latin Education). ABLE is a "street academy," i.e., a school run by and for ghetto people in a store-front operation.

Fortunately, we had wide press and television coverage, which served two purposes. It let addicts know that there was a program for them in their own community. The hundreds of addicts who appeared in our area of the hospital for detoxification and rehabilitation confirmed our worst fears about the depth and breadth of the problem. It also confirmed that we were performing a desperately needed community service. The other purpose was to put the pressure of public opinion against the hospital administration, which made the hospital extremely reluctant to call the police to have us removed and arrested. This not only saved us from jail, but allowed the occupation and thus the program to last longer. We thereby got additional press and television coverage, put more pressure on the hospital, helped to educate the community about their health needs, and developed in them a sense of health consciousness. The recognition that an institution—St. Luke's—in their community—Harlem—was failing to provide needed and relevant services because it had different priorities than the meeting of the community's health needs, developed in the community a considerable degree of awareness. The second purpose was that as the community became galvanized as a result of media coverage, the hospital felt increasingly pressured to meet the community's demand for addiction services.

While the hospital was not pressured or threatened directly by the presence of those who had seized part of it, they were pressured by what the occupiers represented—an enraged, exploited, and explosive community literally up in arms, getting itself together, forming viable coalitions to take on and take over negligent institutions. Plainclothes police did manage to infiltrate the occupied area. However, in view of the hospital's location one block from Harlem, the power relationships between the hospital and the community and those who represented it in the occupation, were more than equalized, thus leading to "rational and reasonable" and relatively prompt negotiations.

The hospital's acceptance of some of the community's demands was aided by the likelihood of some federal money to help finance a forty-bed treatment program. The final settlement was an arrangement for forty beds for addiction services, as well as a satellite addiction service building in another part of the community.

What is clear is that years of negotiations and pleading produced no results, other than the occasional admission of a patient who fit into the existing hospital research and teaching priorities. It was only when the community was agressively and politically assertive that it was rewarded with needed services, services which it could rightfully expect and demand from a publicly funded, but privately serving and unaccountable, community institution. If this study can be generalized, one can't depend upon the "good will and reasonableness" of public institutions to meet the needs of the people, no matter how clearly defined and visible those needs are.

Interestingly enough, the hospital, in its final offer to the community, offered to do a community-wide survey of the community's addiction problem. To the community, who daily experienced and understood the depth of the problem, such a survey was superfluous at best and at worst inflated the cost of health care (if only minimally) by providing a rationalization for a funding grant to the hospital for still more unnecessary or irrelevant research. It hardly matters to the community whether, for example, 10.3 per cent of its members were addicted or 13.8 per cent. To the community and any outside observer the problems were overwhelming, and whatever solutions were offered would in all likelihood be grossly inadequate, in spite of any survey.

One of the major reasons for the continuing and rapid increase in the number of addicts is the need for the criminal market constantly to expand. Addicts themselves attempt to addict other nonaddicts to whom they can sell heroin in order to support their own habit. Such would not be the case if heroin were legalized. Elimination of the black market and criminality would remove the need to expand existing markets and to create new addicts.

Another possible area where we might find some answers is in community/consumer control of all health services, especially those which are publicly funded, which are about 90 per cent of the health facilities in the city. As we have seen currently in the city, the fight for community control of health facilities is being led by such groups as the Black Panthers and the Young Lords, assisted, for example, by the Medical Liberation Front. Already over a hundred community people have been arrested in seizures of health facilities and disruptions of health agency meetings. More is sure to follow as the city's health crisis in general, and addiction problem in particular, worsens.

Well, what is the role of the white professional such as myself in all of this? It is true that in the short run the doctor might be able to see and treat more patients if he does nothing but see and treat them. In the long run, however, he does very little, and by his practice supports both the existing health and political system, both of which are responsible for, and at least in large part the cause of, the very ills the physician is trying to treat, cure, or prevent. Health care is never delivered in a political vacuum. It is either part of the solution or part of the problem.

The gaining of an additional forty beds for addiction services might save more lives and alleviate more disease than a single physician might do in his entire professional lifetime, as simply a doctor in an office or clinic. While the physician, himself, cannot seize or occupy a hospital, he can render a service to the community in a radical context; the physician-patient or physician-community relationship must always be that of equals, open and consultative, where option and alternatives are clearly delineated, where health technology and the profession are demonopolized, demystified and deprofessionalized. Professionalization, mystification, and monopolization of skills through licensing and accrediting procedures are all mechanisms of the existing health and political system to limit services and to channelize the medical market place. Thus any action which exposes this situation is antithetical to the existing health and political system.

It follows that any medical program worth its salt must function so as to challenge the system, raise people's consciousness, and attain by and for them new powers—all the power. Existing health services in many ways do just the opposite, that is, they tend to make do with the limited resources available. If there are overwhelming numbers of people to be served, a program must be designed and the resources allocated to serve them. If the resources can not or will not be allocated, the professional must so inform every member of the community he is in contact with, and not be part of a conspiracy of silence. The community must organize itself to see that it gets these services or at least understands in clear political terms why it doesn't and what it can do to get them. The disparity between what the community comes to realize are its legitimate needs and what it actually gets is the basis of a politicalization process. For the health worker to design a program which lowers the visibility of these needs by fitting the program to mesh with existing and already allocated resources is to decrease the level of politicalization of the people you hope to serve and is thus self-defeating.

What information and services I could and did offer this community were more along the lines of problem delineation (aside from the transfer of skills for withdrawal). The problem was delineated as follows:

1. The addiction problem is so massive and pervasive that simply educating the community and pleading with the hospital will produce no results.

2. The hospital in their community was a publicly funded hospital and as such must serve and not ignore or exploit the community—that the hospital must meet first its public responsibilities and not its institutional needs.

3. The hospital would not serve the community, because

it wasn't to the hospital's advantage to do so, unless forced by a confrontation.

For those of you who find the idea of seizing a hospital to secure lifesaving services a bit threatening, the end is not in sight. The health crisis is worsening.

APPENDICES

Appendix A

When the Department of Parasitology at Columbia University's College of Physicians and Surgeons distributed its final examination on December 15, 1969, to the medical students, it was met with more than the customary anxiety and hisses. Some radical medical students, fed up with the irrelevance and exploitiveness of their medical education, distributed a "guerilla" or "counter" final examination. Their examination was intended to be more truly educative than the conventional one. While some of the more conservative students responded with righteous indignation to the mock final, the majority felt somewhat enlightened.

Parasitology final exam: Dec. 15, 1969

I. Circle the letter that best completes the sentence:
1. Parasitic diseases occur most commonly among —
   a. ignorant blacks in Africa.
   b. filthy natives in South America.
   c. shifty Orientals in the Far East.
   d. ex-slaves in Mississippi.

2. We Americans —
   a. deserve gratitude for showing them how to cook.
   b. could clean up most of the diseases if the natives weren't so ignorant and stubborn.
   c. know what to do with our feces.
   d. will catch their diseases if we allow too many of them in our country.

3. Parasitologists who work overseas —
   a. are among the most dedicated people in the world.
   b. have done a lot to civilize the pagans.
   c. deserve all the money we get.
   d. all of the above.

4. Students of parasitologists who work overseas —
   a. should recognize that they are in the presence of great men.
   b. should keep their opinions to themselves.
   c. are free to do what they are told to do.
   d. a and b, but not c.

5. Students who don't include parasitic diseases in their differential diagnosis —
   a. will be just like the retarded l.m.d.'s (local M.D.)
   b. won't be able to beat the Harvard students on the boards.
   c. are the type who collect small, hard stools.
   d. are no better than the ill-tutored technicians.

6. Firestone Rubber Company —
   a. has done great things to Liberia.
   b. deserves all the profits it gets from Liberian rubber plantations.
   c. shows the Africans the American way of life.
   d. provides medical students with a nice place to take an elective.

II. Choose the best modifier:
1. This department tries out new drugs on South Americans (frequently, occasionally, seldom).
2. Alcoa Aluminium is (good, bad, so what?) for the natives of Surinam.
3. If we didn't send parasitologists to Afghanistan, the Russians would be there (quickly, immediately, violently).
4. The world would be (better off, worse off, a nice place to live) if we stopped giving these people something for nothing.

Extra Credit:

Write an essay explaining why we should have community medicine programs in South Korea and Puerto Rico but not Washington Heights.

Good luck in the pratie of medi$ine!

Appendix B

PREPARED BY DEPT. OF HEW (1970)
COMPARISON OF FIVE PROPOSALS FOR NATIONAL HEALTH INSURANCE

Subject	Griffiths Bill	Committee for National Health Insurance
GENERAL APPROACH	Government universal health insurance program financed by payroll tax and general revenues.	Government universal health insurance program financed by payroll tax and general revenues.
COVERAGE	U.S. residents.	U.S. residents.
BENEFITS	Comprehensive health benefits. Major exclusion is dental services for adults. No cost-sharing except for physician, dentist, and other ambulatory services. ($2 co-pay per visit, with certain exceptions.)	Comprehensive health benefits. Major exclusion is dental services for adults. Limitations on drugs and nursing-home and mental health care. No cost-sharing.
ADMINISTRATION	Federal board composed of HEW officials and nongovernment members; regional offices; advisory bodies.	Federal board under Department of HEW; regional offices; advisory bodies.

COMPARISON OF FIVE PROPOSALS FOR NATIONAL HEALTH INSURANCE

Subject	Griffiths Bill	Committee for National Health Insurance
PAYMENT OF PROVIDERS	*Physician and dentist groups* can contract to receive predetermined payment and pay their members as they choose (including fee for service). *Individual primary physicians and dentists* may elect per capita, salary, or combination of methods and receive an allowance to pay for services of specialists and other health professionals. *Hospitals:* Negotiated budget that includes allowance for nursing-home and home health services.	*Physicians and dentists:* Regional funds allocated first to those in group practice or selecting capitation, salary, or per session basis. Residual allocated to local payment authorities to pay those selecting fee-for-service or per case basis. *Hospitals, nursing homes, home health agencies:* negotiated budget designed to pay reasonable cost under efficient organization.
FINANCING	Tax equal to 7 per cent of payroll, including 1 per cent on employees, 3 per cent on employers, and a payment from general revenues equal to 3 per cent. Earnings base of $15,000, adjusted automatically to increases in wage levels.	Tax equal to about 7¾ per cent (on 1969 basis) including 2.8 per cent on employers, 1.8 per cent on employees and on nonwage income, and general revenues payment equal to 3.1 per cent. Tax levied on first $15,000 of employees and nonwage income combined, and on total payroll for employers.
COST	Cost would have been $35.8 billion in fiscal 1969, according to AFL-CIO.	Cost would have been $37 billion in fiscal 1969, according to CNHI.

COMPARISON OF FIVE PROPOSALS FOR NATIONAL HEALTH INSURANCE

Javits Bill	AMA Medicredit	Pettengill Proposal
Government universal health insurance program (similar to Medicare) with option of "electing out" by purchase of private insurance.[1]	Income tax credits to offset cost of qualified private health insurance.[2]	Private insurance for poor or related groups through an insurance pool subsidized by government.[3]
U.S. residents.	U.S. residents (voluntary).	Poor, near poor, and uninsurables (voluntary).
Same as Medicare (hospital, physician, nursing home, etc.—subject to cost-sharing and limitations). Also, annual check-ups, limited drugs, and dental care for children under age 8.	To be qualified, policy must include basic hospital and physician benefits, and may optionally offer supplementary drug, blood, hospital, and other benefits. Benefits subject generally to cost-sharing and limitations.	Statewide uniform benefits. Minimum benefits to be specified in federal law and to include ambulatory and institutional care.
Department of HEW (as under Medicare) or, under contract with HEW, by state government. Processing of claims conducted by private carriers (as under Medicare) or, under certain conditions, by special quasi-government organizations.	Federal advisory board (including HEW, IRS, and nongovernment members) to establish federal standards for use by state insurance departments in approving private insurance plans.	Statewide insurance pool administered by carrier selected by state with concurrence of federal government.

COMPARISON OF FIVE PROPOSALS FOR NATIONAL HEALTH INSURANCE

Javits Bill	AMA Medicredit	Pettengill Proposal
Until July 1, 1973, reasonable cost for hospital and institutions and reasonable charges for physicians (as under Medicare). Thereafter, new methods, developed in interim, may be employed.	Present methods under private insurance.	Present methods under private insurance.
Tax equal to 10 per cent of payroll, including 3.3 per cent on employers and 3.3. per cent on employees and payment from general revenues equal to 3.3 per cent. Tax levied on $15,000 earnings base for employees and on total payroll for employers.	Financed from federal general revenues.	Poor would pay no premium and the near poor and uninsurables would pay part of the premium. State and federal general revenues would finance the balance of the cost of the program.
Cost of $66.4 billion in 1975, according to Social Security actuary.	Net cost for 1970 estimated at $8 billion by AMA and at $15 billion by SSA.	Estimates not available.

[1] Participants in approved employer-employee health plans and persons purchasing approved private insurance may remain outside of government plan and be exempted from payroll taxes.

[2] Liability on tax return. The maximum (100 per cent) credit would be an amount equal to the premium cost of a qualified health insurance policy.

[3] Proposal also provides (a) a catastrophic protection plan, geared to family income, for the general population, and (b) encouragement for additional coverage under employment-related health insurance.

APPENDIX C

The Patients Association

Do you believe that the medical and nursing services in Great Britain could be greatly improved?

Do you believe that in the past there has been too little respect for the views and emotions of individual patients?

Do you believe that there is a need for an organization to promote and represent the interests of patients?

The Patients Association's objects are:

in all fields of medicine and allied spheres
to represent and further the interests of patients
to provide assistance and advice to patients
to acquire and disseminate information
to promote understanding and goodwill between patients and
all persons engaged in medical practice and related activities.

196

The Patients Association is independent

It depends for funds upon its members. It has no ties—financial or otherwise—with government, the medical profession, or the pharmaceutical industry.

The Patients Association is the only organization solely devoted to promoting and protecting the interest of patients generally. THE PATIENTS ASSOCIATION is non-political, non-profit-making

The Patients Association is democratic

Its Committee is elected by the members, and the Association's policy is thus in the hands of its members. Any member of the Association is eligible for a place on the Committee.

The Patients Association is representative

It represents and furthers the interests of all patients, both in and out of hospital. The Association expresses the points of view of the patient—

in the press and on television and radio

in representations to the Ministry of Health and M.Ps.

in speaking at public and professional meetings

in contacts with the national organisations which represent doctors, nurses and others.

The Patients Association helps

The PATIENTS ASSOCIATION examines complaints and makes enquiries and representations where necessary. It answers queries of all kinds relating to the health services and gives information and advice. It publishes leaflets to assist and inform patients. These include:—

A guide to the Rights of a Patient

Changing your Doctor under the National Health Service

Information and Advice on going into Hospital

Some lesser known Services and Concessions available under the
National Health Service
Compulsory Admission to and Detention in Mental Hospitals
The Association issues a Newsletter to keep its members up to
date about its activities and information of interest to
patients.

The Patients Association finds out

The Association analyses the reports received from patients,
their complaints, criticisms, praise and constructive suggestions. It learns their needs and problems and what improvements are required. It carries out objective surveys into
conditions affecting patients.

The Patients Association is constructive

The Association aims to promote goodwill between patients
and those to whom they turn for healing. Patients are people. Like doctors, they have feelings, emotions, hopes and
fears. It is not just skilled medical and nursing care which
they need when they are sick. Too often patients are made
to feel that they are mere cases, not human beings. Many of
the complaints made about the medical services, especially
in hospital, are attributable to the out-moded attitudes of
some doctors, nurses and administrative staff.
The Patients Association aims to improve the relationship between the medical profession and patients.

The Patients Association is effective

The Association has achieved successes in many fields including—
hospital complaints
hospital visiting
drug safety
human experimentation
the use of patients as teaching material

The Patients Association needs members

The association is a national organization with members in every part of Great Britain. The influence which the Association can bring to bear—both at a national and at a local level—depends directly on the size of its membership. You don't have to be a patient to be a member. If you are in sympathy with the aims of the Association please complete the attached application form and—

become a member of the Patients Association

Index